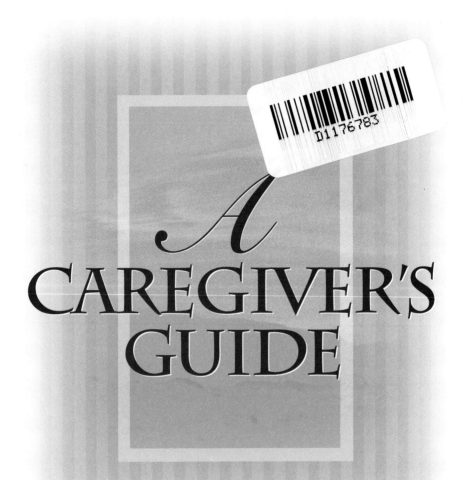

A CAREGIVER'S GUIDE

A *handbook about end of life care*

Karen Macmillan   *Jacquie Peden*
Jane Hopkinson   *Dennie Hycha*

Published by
The Palliative Care Association of Alberta
and
The Military and Hospitaller Order of St. Lazarus of Jerusalem

Canadian Cataloguing in Publication Data:
Macmillan, Karen
    A caregiver's guide: a handbook about end of life care

    Includes bibliographic references and index.
    ISBN: 0-9686700-0-8

    1. Terminally ill-Home care-Handbooks,
manuals, etc. I. Peden, Jacquie II. Hycha, Dennie III .
Hopkinson, Jane H. (Jane Hopkinson) IV.
Hospitaliers of St. Lazarus of Jerusalem. Grand Priory
in Canada V. Palliative Care Association of Alberta
VI. Title

R726.8M32 2000   649.8   C00-900282-0

To contact the authors, write or call:

The Palliative Care Association of Alberta
214-9768 170th Street
Edmonton, AB T5T 5L4
Phone: (780) 447-3980

A Caregiver's Guide will be given to family caregivers at no charge by their regional
health authority home care or palliative care programs. Others may purchase this
book from the Palliative Care Association of Alberta at a cost of $25.00 (including
GST, Shipping and Handling).

Cover, design, layout and illustrations by Robert Weidemann
Printed and bound in Canada by Transcontinental Printing.

Dedication

A Caregiver's Guide

is dedicated to those Albertans

assisting their friends and loved ones

on their final journey.

We hope this book

will help them.

"Be near me when my light is low"
In Memoriam
Alfred, Lord Tennyson

The Development of A Caregiver's Guide

A joint project of the Palliative Care Association of Alberta and the Military and Hospitaller Order of St. Lazarus, A Caregiver's Guide is the result of contributions and review from family care givers and numerous Albertan palliative care professionals in the fields of nursing, medicine, social work, pharmacy, nutrition, physiotherapy, occupational therapy and pastoral counselling. It is designed to assist family caregivers by complementing the guidance and assistance they receive from palliative care and home care professionals.

Over a 12-month period, suggestions for the design, form and content of A Caregiver's Guide were received from palliative care workers across the province. A team of experienced palliative care professionals and health educators reviewed, compiled and wrote A Caregiver's Guide based on this input. After extensive internal review, draft copies were sent back to both palliative care professionals and lay caregivers on two occasions; this final product results from the careful consideration of their responses. We truly appreciate their whole-hearted support and involvement for this important project.

The contributors and reviewers are far too numerous to mention but, for the most part, are either involved with supporting or providing palliative care services through the following Alberta health regions:

• Chinook	• Westview	• Mistahia
• Palliser	• Crossroads	• Peace
• Headwaters	• David Thompson	• Keeweetinok Lakes
• Calgary	• Capital Health	• Northern Lights
• Region 5	• Aspen	• Northwestern
• East Central	• Lakeland	• Alberta Cancer Board

Karen MacMillan and Jacquie Peden compiled the first draft as nurse consultants for the Capital Health Regional Palliative Care Program.

Publication Committee

The publication committee comprised individuals with a cross-section of skills and experience in a variety of palliative care and health education areas. They include:

Dennie Hycha, RN, MN   Publication and Editorial Co-Chair

A palliative care instructor in the Grant MacEwan College Palliative Care Program, Dennie Hycha has clinical experience in palliative care in rural home care, as a staff nurse on an oncology unit and as a clinical instructor of students on an oncology/palliative care unit. Currently the chairperson of the Palliative Care Association of Alberta, her graduate education focused on clinical palliative care.

Robert W. Clarke, CD   Publication and Editorial Co-Chair

Currently the publisher of Family Health magazine, Robert Clarke has had an extensive career in all aspects of Canada's magazine publishing industry. Since founding Family Health in 1985, he has been involved in a variety of health promotion and health education programs and strategies. He is also Commander of the Edmonton Commandery of the Order of St. Lazarus and has served on the Order's national executive for the past five years.

Carleen Brenneis, RN, MHSA   Editorial Adviser

The program director of the Regional Palliative Care Program, Capital Health Authority, Carleen Brenneis's nursing background is in the area of cancer and palliative care. She is presently a member of the Palliative Care Working Group for the Canadian Strategy for Cancer Control.

Jane Hopkinson, BN, MN   Editor

Jane Hopkinson's nursing experience spans 40 years. For her graduate degree, she analyzed vocabulary in health education writing. Since 1985, she has used this knowledge to work as a writer and editor of health information for both the public and health care professions, primarily for the Government of Alberta and Family Health magazine. She is a member of the American Medical Writers Association and has a Certificate in Writing and Editing from that organization.

Karen Macmillan, RN, BScN   Writer

Karen Macmillan has been involved with palliative care in a variety of nursing roles over the past 12 years. She is currently the Community Assessment Nurse for the Tertiary Palliative Care Unit at the Grey Nun's Community Hospital and Health Centre. Her experience includes assistance with Grant MacEwan College's Palliative Care Certificate Program and she has recently completed a certificate in Adult and Continuing Education through the Faculty of Extension at the University of Alberta.

Jacquie Peden, RN, MN   Writer

Having worked in a variety of settings as a nurse over the past 25 years, Jacquie Peden's recent experience includes providing home-based care to the terminally ill. Currently associated with Grant MacEwan Community College as an instructor in the Palliative Certificate Program, she is also self-employed as a nurse consultant in East Central Health Region as the program leader for palliative care and as a contract manager with a project to provide Internet education and information to physicians and nurses working in palliative care.

Edna McHutchion, PhD   Adviser

Currently an associate professor emeritus at the University of Calgary, Edna McHutchion is the former associate dean of the U of C Graduate Program in Nursing. She has an extensive background in the practice of palliative care nursing and is a former president of the Canadian Palliative Care Association.

Pam Berry Otfinowski, RN, BA, BScN   Adviser

With an education in cultural health research and nursing, Pam Berry Otfinowski has previously worked as both a clinical nurse and a research nurse in a variety of palliative care settings. Currently she is a program co-ordinator for the Alberta Cancer Board's Palliative Care Network Initiative which works with regions to help them optimize their existing palliative care programs and services.

Norman Sande, BEd, MEd   Adviser

After 34 years of experience as a high school teacher and administrator, Norman Sande recently retired from the Edmonton Public School Board. He is currently a member of the national council of the Military and Hospitaller Order of St. Lazarus of Jerusalem.

Acknowledgements

We wish to thank and recognize the following individuals, companies and organizations, all of whom played an essential role in the development of *A Caregiver's Guide*:

- Jack and Shirley Singer, United Inc. – Active Living Communities™ and the Alberta Cancer Foundation for their generous financial support without which publication and distribution of *A Caregivers Guide* would not have been possible.

- The Capital Health Authority Regional Palliative Care Program and its medical, nursing and other staff members who so generously supported and contributed to this project.

- Family Health magazine, and especially Cathy Berry, administrative assistant, who throughout the development of this project provided much needed administrative and logistical support, co-ordination of editorial copy flow and other production support.

- The director and members of the Palliative Care Association of Alberta who actively contributed to the planning and review of *A Caregiver's Guide*.

- The members of the Calgary and Edmonton Commanderies of The Order of St. Lazarus who, in so many ways, supported the publication of this book.

- The valuable contributions from Rob Weidemann with the design, layout and illustration of *A Caregiver's Guide*.

We wish to recognize the many palliative care and home care professionals whose mission is to help their fellow Albertans through this difficult stage of life.

Dennie Hycha
President
Palliative Care Association of Alberta

Robert Clarke
Commander, Edmonton
Order of St. Lazarus

Table of Contents

Introduction

Understanding Palliative Care

As you take care of someone with a terminal illness, you are facing what many describe as one of the toughest, but possibly most rewarding challenges of life. It is not going to be easy. Although you may not be able to stop your loved one from dying, you can help to make the last days more comfortable. Care at this stage of life is called palliative care or hospice care.

The World Health Organization, in its definition of palliative care, states that the goal is "to provide the best possible quality of life for patients and their families." To achieve this, palliative care:

- views dying as an inevitable part of life.
- does not bring on nor delay death.
- provides relief from pain and other distressing symptoms.
- covers all aspects of care, including physical, psychological, social, emotional and spiritual issues.
- offers a support system to help patients live as actively as possible until death.
- provides support to the family coping with the loved one's illness and during grief after death.
- respects personal, cultural, lifestyle and religious values and beliefs.

A caregiver can be a family member or friend who is available to care for the dying person. The care may also be provided by a group of people. The choice to provide palliative care can be difficult to make. You need to consider many factors including your health and your ability both physically and emotionally to provide the care. You also need to take into account your previous relationship with the person. Providing the care may mean you need to take time off work and this may be a major decision for you.

Being a caregiver in the home can be physically and emotionally stressful. However you do not need to do it alone. There is support offered by the health care team in your area. A team approach with you as a key member is often the best way to provide care in the home. This team may consist of the family doctor, home care nurse, other health care workers, a pastor or spiritual adviser, volunteers, other family members, and friends. With a team approach the physical, emotional, psychological and spiritual needs of the ill person and the family can be met in the best way.

This team helps provide care as well as support for you. You need to share your concerns or cultural and spiritual practices with the team members so your needs are met. They can help you and your loved one to cope with the issues and stages of the dying process, and try to make this final journey of life the best experience possible.

Even when you have committed yourself, you will need breaks from the caregiving role. This may be just a few minutes to go for a walk, read a book, or talk to a friend. Always remember that changing your mind about your decision to be a caregiver at a later date is okay.

Most family caregivers say that getting the right information is one of their most important needs in providing palliative care in the home. This handbook was developed to provide that information. To get the most from it read it when you need information on a certain topic. Discuss anything you do not understand with your health care worker. If you read the whole book, remember that all parts may not apply to you. Each person is different and may experience illness in a different way.

There are some points to bear in mind about the use of this handbook.
- Medical words that might not be understood have all been explained. The pages where these explanations can be read are indicated in the Index.
- The handbook has a lay-flat binding so you can open it flat at any page without fear of damage.
- Throughout, suggestions have been made for brand name products available for dealing with particular problems. This list is not complete and many similar products work just as well. Ask your pharmacist for advice. Any mention of specific brands does not mean the developers of this guide endorse this product.

Contact Names and Numbers

Throughout the guide under the heading Important Points it has been suggested that you call for help about specific things. The information about whom to call has not been included because each person's needs are different. Often it means that you need to call your home care nurse. Ask a member of your health care team to help you note whom you should call for a particular concern. A list of some of these with a space to fill in their telephone numbers, is found on the next page. You might find it helpful to photocopy this page so you can keep it in a prominent place. There are also a blank pages at the end of the book where you can make notes about your specific needs and people who can help you.

	Name	Number
Family doctor		
Home care coordinator		
Home care nurse		
Physiotherapist		
Occupational therapist		
Social worker		
Support worker/Homemaker		
Volunteer		
Pastor or spiritual advisor		
Pharmacist		
Respiratory therapist		
Respiratory equip. vendor		
Dietitian		
Family and friends		
Other contacts:		

When a terminal illness is first diagnosed

COMING TO TERMS WITH WHAT IS HAPPENING

When someone very close to you has a terminal illness, the adjustment is extremely difficult. It usually takes a long time and a lot of effort to come to terms with what is happening. For everyone involved there is a very normal sense of approaching change and loss. These feelings usually bring about a reaction called anticipatory grief.

During this time, as a caregiver you may find that:

- time stands still.
- priorities change.
- life and death take on new meanings.
- things you previously took for granted are changed forever.
- your hopes for the future are gone.
- life may even lose its meaning for a while.

WHAT YOU AND YOUR LOVED ONE MAY EXPECT

The knowledge that death is not far away colours all aspects of living.

- Shock, numbness, disbelief, panic, helplessness and hopelessness are common.
- You may have thoughts of all the losses and changes you have faced, as well as current and future ones. These include family roles, control over life events, body image, sexual feelings, financial changes, future hopes and dreams.
- In your anxiety you may have increased fears relating to death, uncontrollable pain and suffering.
- Your emotions may seem as if they are on a roller-coaster.
- There will be times when you deny what is happening and other moments when everything seems too much to bear.
- You may sometimes think that others do not seem to care as much as you do.
- Anger, sadness, guilt and blame can seem overwhelming.
- There may be periods of questioning "Why did this happen to me?"

These feelings may go on for weeks and change day to day, hour to hour. As you grieve each new loss, it may seem as if you are in a dream from which you hope you will soon wake.

- All these reactions are normal.
- Each person's grief before and after a death is very personal and must unfold in its own time and in its own way.
- There are no set ways or quick fixes to help you through, but there are some things that may help.

HOW YOU CAN HELP
YOUR LOVED ONE AND YOURSELF

If you and your loved one share anticipatory grief, you may be able to support one another and take comfort from special moments together.

- Take your cues from how your loved one is feeling, but acknowledge your feelings as well. Keeping a daily journal may help you to do this.
- Be truthful, especially when you or your loved one is doing poorly. Everyone, whether sick or well, should be treated with honesty.
- Respect the privacy of the sick person and allow as much control as possible when making decisions about care and activities.
- Go easy on giving advice and be open to its being ignored.
- Share your hopes, thoughts and feelings with your loved one. It may provide comfort to you both, and build a better understanding of what is important and how you can provide the best support.
- Enjoy the good days and make the best of your times together. This can be a good time for you and your loved one to share special moments and remember the important things in your lives. It may help you both adjust to what is happening.
- Reminisce about your life together, the good and the not so good.
- Include your loved one in family activities whenever possible.
- Spend time together talking, listening to music, watching television, playing cards or games. Share your thoughts and feelings, laughter and tears.
- Try to resolve any conflicts or unfinished business that you might have. If this is difficult, perhaps a third person can help both of you come to an understanding.
- Share your plans for the future, even though it seems impossible to imagine.
- Help the person with putting affairs in order. Settling the estate can help you both to prepare. This is a good time to check that your loved one's will is up to date and you know where it is.

- Take care of yourself. Talk about your feelings and concerns with someone you trust and who understands your situation such as a family member, friend, counsellor or religious adviser.
- Keep important family routines and let the others go for a while.
- Know and accept your limits. You cannot provide all the answers, solve all the problems or provide all the care. Accept help from others who want to be involved.

WHAT YOU MIGHT EXPECT AS YOUR LOVED ONE GETS SICKER

As the illness progresses, both you and your loved one will have many changing emotions.

- Increasing fear, yearning, anxiety, edginess, irritability and sadness may occur.
- You may both feel totally out of control, confused and powerless.
- Mood swings between periods of denial and acceptance, hopefulness and hopelessness are common.
- The person who is dying may withdraw from normal life activities.
- Changing physical appearance may make the person reluctant to be seen by others.
- The person may become anxious about being a burden.
- At times you may be uncertain about what you should be doing.
- You may become distracted causing you to wonder if your memory is poor.
- Worries about how you will cope now and after the death may be present.
- You may have a greater awareness of your own mortality.

IMPORTANT POINTS

- Do not tell a sad person to "cheer up" as this just creates further anxiety and distance.
- **Call for help if:**
  - *fear, anxiety or sadness are severe, or go on for several days, or the person expresses thoughts of suicide.*
  - *the person refuses to eat, cannot sleep or takes no interest in daily activities.(Bear in mind that these may be normal in the last days of life but may indicate a need for help at this stage.)*
  - *feelings of guilt, worthlessness and hopelessness are strong.*
  - *the person complains of being unable to breathe, is sweating or is very restless, because these may be symptoms of anxiety.*
  - *you are tired and need relief.*

CARING FOR YOURSELF – THE CAREGIVER

Caring for your loved one who is ill can be rewarding but it can also be physically and emotionally draining. It is difficult to predict how long you will be providing the care. If you are going to keep giving to others, you must make sure that you take care of yourself as well.

WHAT YOU CAN DO TO CARE FOR YOURSELF

Keeping healthy

Although a terminal illness is happening to a loved one, the entire family is affected. When you first start to care for your loved one at home, there may be a temptation to feel you must meet the needs of everyone around you. Some common sense ideas for easing the workload and caring for yourself tend to be overlooked.

- Prepare proper meals for your family and eat on a regular schedule even when it seems you are too tired or too busy.
- Prepare double portions when you cook so you have a second meal in the freezer.
- Stock up on healthy snacks such as fruit or cheese and whole grain crackers for those times you are very busy but need to eat.
- Make time for a regular schedule of exercise.
- Keep up with your regular dental and medical appointments.
- Plan to sleep when the person sleeps if you are tired.
- Ask someone to relieve you so you can have an unbroken eight hours of sleep if you are short of sleep several days in a row.
- Do not fret if the household chores are not done to your usual standard. If you can arrange it, hire someone to do the heavy work such as vacuuming and laundry. This type of help may be available through home care or other community services. Ask your home care nurse.
- If you have an outside job, consider taking a leave of absence if possible.

Coping skills

Caring for someone with a terminal illness takes its toll on you mentally as well as physically. It is normal to be despairing, angry and frustrated but the way you manage those feelings will make a difference to how you feel after your loved one has died.

- Call on family or friends to help you when the load seems too heavy. They can help with tasks such as making meals, sitting with the person or baby-sitting.
- Take the chance for a break when you need it, and do not feel guilty about it. At work, your breaks can be your job when you can concentrate on something other than the person you are caring for.
- Remember that others are on edge and also trying to cope so try to see things from their point of view when tense situations arise.
- Break big problems down into manageable size by working at them one step at a time.
- Set realistic goals for yourself for the amount you are able to do.
- Try to set aside special time for the other loved ones in your life, even if it means scheduling it into your day.

Managing your emotions

For some people, the experience of providing palliative care intensifies the love for the dying person. Sometimes there is a feeling of increased inner strength and resolve. For everyone, feelings of sadness, anger, fear and anxiety are normal in times of stress. You may feel up one day and down the next. You may be sad and angry at the same time. You may fear the loss of your loved one, anger at why this person has to die, frustration at not being able to "do enough" or stress due to increased responsibility at home. Remember there is no right way to feel at this time.

- Find ways to blow off steam. Try a round of vigorous exercise, pounding a pillow, or sitting alone in a car and screaming - anything that works to relieve the tension.
- Get resentment off your chest. If you need a sounding board, talk to a friend, family member, or professional.
- Find a support group where you can talk with others who have been in your position and understand your feelings. Your home care nurse can tell you about groups in your region.
- Consider discussing your situation with a member of your health care team if your relationship with the person is affected by a history of abuse, addiction or conflict. You may have serious problems giving the care.
- Seek the help of your spiritual or religious adviser if this will help you.

- Avoid, if you can, people or situations that make you angry.
- Step away from the situation if you feel your frustration rising, before you say something in the heat of the moment.
- Cry if that helps. It is a normal reaction and a good way of coping.
- Laugh without feeling guilty. It is a good way of releasing tension.
- Write your experiences in a journal as a way of releasing your emotions.
- Practice deep breathing and relaxation techniques.
- Pat yourself on the back for all that you have done.
- Ask your home care nurse about the possibility of counselling if you think that would help.

Respite care

People in the health care profession often use the word respite (pronounced "res-pit"). It means "rest." Respite is taking a break from the responsibilities of being a caregiver. It can help you feel refreshed and better able to cope whether you physically leave home or not. The length of the break depends how comfortable you feel being away.

- Ask a friend or family member to care for your loved one while you go.
- Speak to your home care nurse who may be able to organize respite care.
- Your loved one can be admitted into a bed in a long term care setting or hospice for a short time to give you a break.
- Helpers can go into the home to stay with the person. They may:
  - come in at night to keep the person company.
  - give food or drinks to the person.
  - help the person to move about in bed.
  - just stay close by to allow caregivers time to take care of themselves.
  - Explain to your loved one that you need the extra help to keep providing the care at home.
- Try taking physical breaks by:
  - going for a walk.
  - working in your garden.
  - sitting in your backyard.
  - going for lunch with a friend.
  - going to a movie.
  - finding a restful place and being in the quiet.

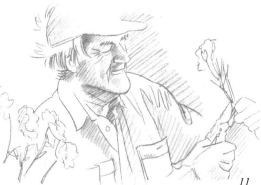

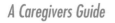

- Try taking mental breaks by:
  - meditating.
  - reading a book.
  - listening to music you enjoy.
  - watching television.
  - doing handicrafts.
  - talking to a friend.
- Nourish your spirit by engaging in any spiritual activity that comforts you.

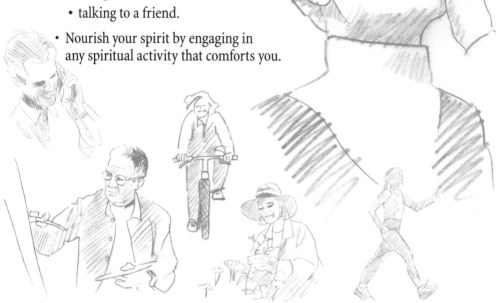

IMPORTANT POINTS

Caregiver "Burnout"

The word "burnout" describes the exhaustion of physical or emotional strength. It is a good description of the way you may feel sometimes. Seek help from some in your support network if you find that any of the following are happening.

- The urge to run and hide from responsibility becomes strong.
- Your activity is scattered and frantic.
- There is a major change in your sleeping patterns or eating habits.
- You are often irritable or easily angered.
- Important details are forgotten or you cannot concentrate.
- You use alcohol, drugs or tobacco more than before.
- You lose more than 10 pounds, or sleep less than three hours, or cannot read more than a few sentences without losing concentration.

Remember, often a few hours for yourself is all you need to keep going.

SUPPORT NETWORKS

The care of a dying person is not easy and requires a team of people with different skills and ideas. You are a key part of this team. Other team members are there to help both you and your loved one. This is a network that includes informal support from family and friends and formal support from the health care team.

INFORMAL SUPPORT

To organize your support group, identify who may be willing or who has offered to help. Sometimes this help can come from unexpected sources and be prepared for the possibility that some family and friends whom you think will be helpful do not want to become involved.

- Make a list of what you need done and post it prominently. Visitors do not know your routine and may hesitate to ask but would be willing to do tasks such as change the cat litter or do laundry if they knew those were needed. Review and update your list on a regular basis.
- Ask for help. Most people want to help so let them know how.
- Enlist the help of someone to screen calls and provide information.
- Request practical help with tasks such as shopping, making meals and housework.
- Find out when people are available to help.
- Some people to ask for help are:
  - family, friends, neighbours.
  - members from your social organizations or faith community.
  - minister, priest or other religious or spiritual advisers.
- Find out those who may be willing to:
  - listen to your concerns.
  - sit with the person while you take a break.
  - make a meal, do the laundry, mow the lawn, shovel the walks.
  - pick up a prescription or drive you to an appointment.
- Your community may have volunteers who will visit to read aloud, play cards, provide transportation or any other support you need.

FORMAL SUPPORT

Your formal support network is more structured than the informal one. It may include:

- family doctor who is willing to visit the person at home.

- home care nurse.

- other members of the home care team such as occupational therapists, physiotherapists, social workers, respiratory therapists and volunteers.

- personal care workers or home support aides who provide care and can give the caregivers a break.

- pharmacist at your drugstore who will deliver medications to your home and will provide information about medications.

- dietitian.

- community agencies that offer useful services from volunteers or for a fee. These include meals, house cleaning, grocery shopping, shovelling walks or mowing the lawn.

IMPORTANT POINTS

- Support networks are there to help you and your loved one but you may need to be specific about what you need at that time.
- Remember that help is available. Do not try to do everything yourself.
- Make lists of questions and concerns about the person's care as they occur. Have them in front of you when you talk with friends and the health care team.
- Having helpers in the home always takes some getting used to. Even visits from members of the health care team such as nurses or personal care workers will need some adjustment by all the family.

- You may ask your family doctor for help contacting home care or you may telephone them yourself. Someone from home care will come out to your home and assess the needs of you and your loved one. The type of support and services that are provided depend on what is available in the region where you live.

- All home care programs have nurses but some may not include all the professionals listed above.

- Home care programs may provide different services in different locations. Additional services may include:
  - giving advice about the person's symptoms and health related problems.
  - providing emotional support to you and your loved one.
  - visiting to determine what you or the person needs.
  - bathing, feeding or moving the person.
  - staying with the person while you take a break.
  - referrals to other community agencies.

- If your loved one is resisting help from others, explain that you need the help and would like to give the service a try.
- Financial help from several sources may be available (see Appendix I, p.130). This may be a good time to learn what you will need to know about the person's financial affairs such as the locations of bank accounts, mortgages, investments, charge cards and a will.

EFFECTIVE COMMUNICATION WITH OTHERS

COMMUNICATING WITH YOUR LOVED ONE

Communication involves talking, listening and the "gift of presence." This means simply being with a person and listening in a sympathetic way. Remember that touching, holding, hugging and caressing are ways to express the acceptance and caring that may be so important. More than words, they show your ongoing love for the person. This may be a chance to enrich your relationships with both your loved one and other family members.

How you can offer care

Your loved one may be experiencing many emotions such as fear, anxiety and anger. You can be a great support by being an active and interested listener.

- Squeeze a hand or offer an embrace to show how much you care. Sitting in silence can be as supportive as conversation.
- Smile and laugh at humorous incidents and happy memories. Do not let illness put a ban on laughter.
- Continue to enjoy things together that have meaning such as music, art, sports, movies or books on tape.

- Help the person you are caring for to stay in contact with friends and outside activities by assisting with letter-writing, phone calls and visits.
- Be a sounding board for the person to talk about fears and concerns.
- Talk about your feelings and fears too.
- Be aware that your loved one may be expressing anger by taking it out on you. If this happens often or you find it difficult to cope with this, you may need outside help.
- If the person cannot speak, ask a member of your health care team for ideas such as using a communication board.
- Consider several good books listed on page 124 that may help you as you talk to your loved one. Three in particular are:
  - Buckman, R. (1988). *I don't know what to say.* Toronto, ON: Key Porter Books Limited.
  - Jevne, R. F. (1994). *The voice of hope: heard across the heart of life.* San Diego, CA: LuraMedia.
  - Jevne, R. F. (1991). *It all begins with hope: patients, caregivers & the bereaved speak out.* San Diego, CA: LuraMedia.

Guidelines for talking

- Accept what the person is saying, however different it may be from what you think.
- Clarify anything that is unclear to you so you can be sure you understand what has been said and what it means.
- Share your perceptions and feelings.
- Use "I" statements when communicating your own needs or feelings. An example would be "I want to help but I need you to tell me how."
- Be honest but not hurtful with your comments and observations.
- Encourage but do not push, your loved one to share thoughts and feelings.
- Try different openings for conversation. You could start with an observation like "You seem relaxed (or not relaxed) today." Asking if there is anything the person wants to talk about is also a good way to start a conversation. Give broad openings so the conversation and topic can go many directions.
- Be willing to say you do not know the answers to what will happen in the future.
- Be aware that it is not uncommon for a person to return to the use of an original language as death comes closer. If you do not speak the language, try to find someone who does.

Guidelines for listening

- Pay attention to what is being said, to the tone of voice and body language, as well as the words themselves. A person often has more insight when speaking aloud. Use your listening skills after beginning with openings such as "Tell me more about ..." or "What does it mean to you to ...?"
- Be attentive and try not to let your mind wander to your own thoughts and reactions. Good listening takes concentration.
- Test your understanding by "checking out" what you have just heard. This helps keep things clear.
- Listen carefully for meaningful questions that the person really wants answered. If need be, the question will be repeated. Many questions need no answer but open up areas for discussion.
- Respect what the person chooses to talk about rather than taking the lead yourself. If you follow the mood of the person, you will have no difficulty laughing together over the absurd events of the day or seriously considering some of the mysteries of life.

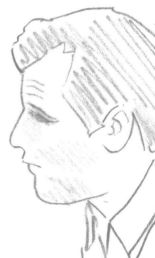

Things to avoid

- Do not make promises you cannot keep and do not fill your loved one with empty reassurances.
- Do not make judgments about what the person says or does. Everyone has a right to an opinion and that right should be respected.
- Do not try to avoid uncomfortable issues by changing the subject or introducing an unrelated topic. Express your discomfort and suggest that the concern be shared with someone else. If you are the only one the person will confide in, you might want to get help dealing with the issue.

COMMUNICATING WITH OTHER FAMILY MEMBERS

When you care for someone with a life threatening illness, you will probably find it helpful to let those close to you offer support. It is comforting to confide your fears and hopes rather than trying to hide them.

How you can offer comfort

- Reminisce as a family to review your lives together. Remember the best and worst moments, family strengths, important times and events.
- Help the person write letters to keep in touch with other family members.
- Keep a scrapbook of your times together. In future years you will be able to look back through photos and mementos.
- Talk about your concerns and encourage others to do the same. Many people who want to talk about their fears are reluctant because they do not want to upset the family. On the other hand respect the fact that the person may not wish to talk about some feelings and thoughts.
- Talk about the future and make important decisions as soon as possible while the dying person can still be included in them.
- Deal with changes in family roles and responsibilities. Ask the person to help you learn to do unfamiliar tasks previously their responsibility.

COMMUNICATING WITH CHILDREN

It is important to give children opportunities to ask questions about a life-threatening illness and to express their feelings.

- Do not try to "spare" your children from knowing that a loved one is dying. Children sense the truth.
- Remember that children have amazing capabilities when they understand a situation. It is whispered conversations behind closed doors that make them imagine situations that are worse than reality.
- Learn what the children understand and their reactions to the situation.
- Include children in activities with the person but never force an issue.

- Keep visits short for small children.
- Let the school know what is happening.
- Reserve time for the children.
- Be consistent in your care of the children.
- Consider some of the excellent books that are available to help you discuss dying with your children. See Books to Help Grieving Children, page 126, for suggestions.

COMMUNICATING WITH THE HEALTH CARE TEAM

You need to communicate with your loved one's doctor, nurse or other member of the health care team. Remember that any final decision about care should rest in the hands of the dying person. Use the advice you get from the health care team as a starting point for discussion.

What you need to consider

- Try to deal with several concerns at one contact. Think about what you need to know and who might be the best person to provide assistance.
- Write down your important questions as you think of them. Also, make note of questions your loved one has, even those mentioned in casual conversation. When it is time to ask the questions, either record the answers yourself or have someone with you to do it.
- Make sure you understand the advice you are given. Ask questions before you hang up or leave the office.
- If you are unsure about the answers or cannot remember, go over your recorded answers later.
- Tell a member of the health care team about new pains or symptoms immediately so attention can be paid to them early.
- Remember that members of the health care team can also help with your emotional and spiritual needs.
- Tell the doctor about other medical or complementary therapies your loved one may be using. This is extremely important as there may be serious side effects.
- Once a decision on treatment is mutually decided, follow the advice but remember that you can ask anytime to discuss the choices you have made.

COMMUNICATING WITH VISITORS

When friends and family know that someone is dying, they want to have a chance to spend some final time with a loved one. There are some basic guidelines you can provide so that you can be sure the person is able to enjoy the visits.

- Talk to the person about visitors and ask if they are tiring. Use this as your guide to decide on the number of visitors and their length of stay.
- Give visitors a limit for the length of their visit.
- Encourage visitors to phone first and tell them if it is not a good time to come.
- Suggest that visitors just sit quietly or talk in a way that does not require an answer if talking causes breathlessness.
- Ask them to visit less often if there are periods when the person seems to tire more easily.
- Discourage anyone from visiting who seems to have a cold or the flu.
- Try using a sign on your front door to indicate when you do not want visitors.
- Consider having a guest book that you can keep to remember all who supported you and your loved one by visiting.

During this time family and friends may be unsure about what they should do.

- Friends wonder if they should visit and for how long.
- They are not sure what to talk about and wonder whether or not to bring up the possibility of death.
- They are uncertain if they should draw closer or pull away from their loved one.
- They wonder whether and when to say their goodbyes.

There are no right or wrong answers. Remember each situation is different. Sometimes it helps to take cues from what the dying person talks about. It is better to do whatever you feel is best "just in case" death occurs sooner than expected. As a caregiver you can only guide visitors according to what seems right at the time.

SPIRITUAL NEEDS

For some people, spirituality is how they see themselves in relation to others, the earth and the universe. For others, a spiritual power is at the heart of these relationships. The spiritual power may be God, Allah, Buddha, Hindu deities or any of the many supreme beings that are worshipped. Those who embrace this type of spirituality often do so within an organized religion. Even within a specific religion there may be some who pray differently and have differing ways of relating to this spiritual power. For these reasons, the spiritual needs of a dying person may be obvious at times and not so obvious at other times. A common spiritual need no matter what a person's belief system is the search for the meaning of life and purpose for living.

What you need to understand

Some people understand or seek meaning for their suffering within the context of their religious belief system. Others look for meaning elsewhere.

- Your loved one may have lost contact with a faith community but want to return.
- Maybe the person wishes to re-establish broken ties with a spiritual power.
- For some, the longing is for a relationship with a previously unknown spiritual power.
- The person may express guilt, remorse and a desire for forgiveness in a search for inner peace and peace with others or a spiritual power.
- Your loved one may ask "Why?" either of the spiritual power or the universe at large. The question may not be asked aloud but suggested by what is being said.
- If prayer has been a big part of your loved one's life, this need for prayer may change. The person may no longer feel the comfort of a close bond with a spiritual power.
- For a religious person there may be deep spiritual anguish either spoken or unspoken, over the perceived absence of a spiritual power. These feelings are not a denial of beliefs but an attempt to understand why this suffering is permitted.
- The person may start to look back on life and look ahead to the unknown. There may be hopes of a miracle or of immortality, either in a life hereafter or a human legacy.

How you can offer comfort

Your role in providing comfort is listening and helping your loved one sort through the varied emotions that accompany a terminal illness.

- Help a loved one who has a need for prayer, to remember that even if prayer does not come easily, others are offering prayers.
- Tell the person's important spiritual supports about the illness and ask them to be available as spiritual companions.
- Do not feel compelled to offer your own answers to any of the searching questions the person asks of a spiritual power.
- Ask the person if it would be helpful to talk to someone about spiritual matters, even if this type of contact has not been important before now. Often the chaplain from the home care team can be helpful.
- Reassure the person that feelings of doubt or guilt can be normal at this time.
- Accept the person's need to talk about dying or saying good-bye.
- Make sure you have your own spiritual resources to help you.

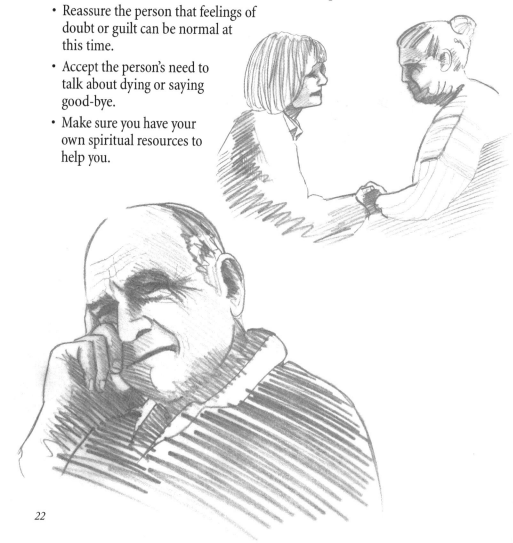

ADAPTING YOUR HOME

What you need to consider

When caring for someone at home, you need to consider where most of the care will be provided.

- Will the person spend most of the time in bed?
- Will the preference be to stay in the bedroom or closer to the family activities?
- Is it necessary to have a bathroom close by?
- Can the person climb stairs?

How you can offer comfort and care

With a few changes to household arrangements, you should be able to adapt your home without too much disruption.

- Avoid having throw rugs on the floor as they slip easily and might cause a fall.
- Create an area, near a window if possible, surrounded by favourite pictures, music and pets.
- Keep helpful items within reach of a comfortable bed. These include:
  - a small table at the height of the bed for medication, snacks, radio, notepaper.
  - a comfortable armchair nearby that is high enough for ease of getting in or out.
  - a foot stool to help the person in and out of a high bed.
  - a small bell, 'baby monitor' or buzzer to call for help.
- Ask your home care nurse about home aids and equipment that can make care at home easier. Many of these can be rented. Examples of home aids and equipment are:

  - hospital bed
  - bed rails (full or half length)
  - rubber sheets
  - overbed table
  - sheepskin (natural or synthetic)
  - alternating pressure mattress
  - bedpan/slipper pan/urinal

  - hot water bottle
  - commode
  - raised toilet seat/toilet arm rest
  - hair washing tray
  - supportive mattress or cushion (e.g. Spenco™)
  - walker
  - wheelchair
  - cane, crutches
  - foam cushion

  - back rest
  - bolster/wedge
  - bath rail
  - bath board
  - bath lift
  - bath chair
  - floor to ceiling pole
  - transfer belt
  - trapeze bar

Giving Physical Care

INFECTION CONTROL (Universal Precautions)

The reason for infection control is that anyone may carry any number of bacteria (germs). Therefore, the rules of precaution apply to everyone. Universal precautions protect you and the person you are caring for from infection. The equipment you may need such as gloves, aprons and masks can be purchased from your pharmacist or a business that sells health supplies. The cost of these may be covered by some programs. Your home care nurse can advise you about this and about the need to use some of the precautions such as gloves and aprons.

Handwashing

Washing your hands is the most effective way to prevent spread of infections. Wash with warm soapy water before and after every contact with the person you are caring for. Prevent dryness and chapping with hand lotion and keep your cuticles and nails trimmed so your hands are easy to keep clean.

Garbage disposal

All dirty dressings or other used, disposable products with blood or body fluids on them must be inside two plastic bags for disposal. This is intended to keep all of the bacteria contained within the bags so they will not spread infection.

Gloves

Disposable latex or vinyl gloves should be worn for handling objects which have blood or body fluids on them. Disposable gloves should never be reused and should be put in the two plastic bags in the garbage.

Aprons

Wear a disposable plastic apron if your clothes are likely to be soiled while you give care. Place the apron in the two plastic bags in the garbage when you take it off.

Masks

Wear a mask if you have a cold. You can protect yourself with a mask when the person you are caring for is coughing a lot.

Needles and syringes

Place used needles and syringes in a hard plastic or metal container that has a lid. Place the lid on the container when it is full and tape it shut so the needles will not fall out and stick anyone. The procedure for disposal varies across the province so ask your home care nurse how it is done in your community.

Food preparation

Raw foods are prime carriers of germs. Meats and eggs should be cooked thoroughly. Fruits and vegetables should always be washed before you cook or eat them. Wash dishes, glassware and cooking utensils in hot, soapy water. If you use a cutting board to prepare raw meat, always wash the board in hot water before you use it again.

Pets

Since animals can carry disease, it is important to make sure that family pets are healthy and up-to-date for check-ups or shots. Make sure you wash your hands thoroughly after you clean the cat's litter box or the bird's cage.

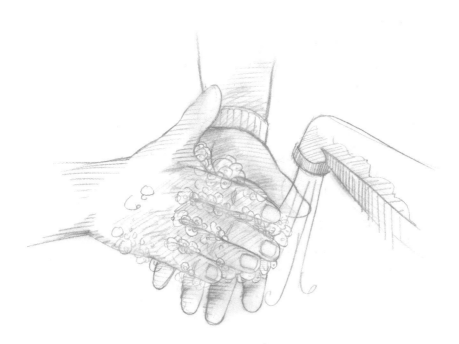

BATHING

Bathing is an important part of personal care and offers both physical and emotional comfort.

How you can offer care

Someone who is strong enough and able to move about can be helped to wash in a shower, bath tub, or at the sink.

- Put a bath chair on a non-slip mat in the tub or shower if getting in and out or standing for a long time is difficult. A chair at the sink can also be used if this seems to work better.
- Ask your home care nurse or occupational therapist for ideas to make the bathroom safer and easier for the person to use. Equipment such as bars for holding, non-slip surfaces and bath lifts may be helpful.
- Gather all the things you will need before helping the person into the bathroom:
  - clean clothes or pyjamas
  - soap and shampoo
  - face cloth
  - towel
  - lotion
- Test the water temperature of the bath or shower.
- Help the person get into the bath or shower.
- Allow the person to wash as much as possible. You may need to help with the back, legs, feet and genital area.
- Offer assistance out of the bath or shower and help to dry. A towel put in the drier for a few minutes before it is needed can provide added warmth.
- Help the person into clean clothes.

BED BATH

Someone who must stay in bed will benefit from a bed bath every day. As well as providing cleanliness, it helps refresh your loved one and gives you the chance to talk and listen.

How you can offer care

Although a bed bath can be given at anytime, often people who are ill have more energy in the morning. Ask the person what time would be best.

- Provide privacy.
- Gather the things you will need:
  - large bowl with warm water
  - soap
  - wash cloth and towels
  - light bed cover
  - lotion

> **IMPORTANT POINTS**
>
> - If movement causes pain, give pain medication about 30 minutes before the bath.
> - Avoid powder as it tends to cake in body creases.
> - Home care help may be available for personal care.

- Raise the level of the bed if this is possible to lessen the strain on your back.
- Cover the person with a light cover for warmth and only uncover and wash one part of the body at a time.
- Use a gentle soap on the skin, then rinse and dry.
- Start at the face and work down towards the feet.
- Apply lotion if desired after drying an area.
- Wash front and sides first, then help the person to lie on one side while you wash the back.
- Wash the genital and anal areas last. It is important that these areas be cleaned well at least daily as bacteria tend to collect there. Wash between the person's legs from the front toward the back. Rinse well.
- Apply a water-repellent cream (e.g. Penaten Cream™, Zincofax™, A&D Cream™) to the genital area if incontinence is a problem.
- Change the water as often as necessary to keep it clean and hot.
- Wash the person's face, hands, back, underarms and genitals daily if a complete bath is too tiring.
- Apply lotion to all pressure areas. Also, while you are using the lotion, the person may appreciate a complete back rub (see Attention to Pressure Areas, p.33).
- Change soiled or wet sheets after the bed bath is finished (see Making a Bed with Someone in it, p.37).
- Remember shaving, make-up and brushing and styling hair are important parts of care and will help the person feel more comfortable. Often a rest before and after these activities will help prevent the person from becoming over-tired.

MOUTH CARE

Cleaning a person's mouth is not difficult. By helping your loved one have a clean mouth you will increase comfort, prevent mouth sores and maybe improve appetite.

How you can offer care

Brushing teeth

- Help the person into a sitting position. If it is more comfortable, or if the person can not sit, help lift the head.
- Place a dry towel under the chin.
- Give the person a sip of water to moisten the inside of the mouth.
- Use an ultra-soft toothbrush and soften the bristles in hot water.
- Do not use toothpaste as it can be harsh on fragile gum tissue. Moisten the brush in one of the rinsing solutions suggested later in this section under Rinsing.
- Brush the teeth using gentle strokes starting at the gumline and moving to the edge of the teeth.
- Brush the cheeks, gums and tongue gently.
- Do not put the toothbrush too near the back of the throat as this may cause gagging.
- Try to remove all food particles and crusted material.
- Have the person rinse with cool water and spit into the bowl or basin.
- If the person is unconscious, use a soft toothbrush moistened in one of the rinsing solutions or a toothette (a swab with a sponge head - see warning under Important Points). Gently rub along the teeth, gums and tongue.

Denture care

- If the person has dentures, remove these and clean them with a toothbrush.
- Do not use very hot water on dentures as they may warp.
- Do not soak dentures in bleach as this may damage them. Any commercially available product marketed for denture soaking may be used.
- If the gums are dry under dentures, a product such as Oral Balance™ may provide comfort.
- If dentures are loose or poor fitting, they may cause mouth sores. Have them refitted by a denturist or, if this is not possible, leave them out except when eating.

Lip care

- Put a water-soluble lubricant such as K-Y Jelly™, Muco™ or Dermabase™ on the lips.
- Avoid using oil-based products such as Vaseline™, Chapstick™ and mineral oil. These may make open sores on the lips more inflamed. Also, if a person is unconscious, an oil-based product may be breathed into the lungs and cause pneumonia.

Rinsing

- Rinsing the mouth is not a substitute for brushing.
- If the person is not able to get out of bed, the mouth should be rinsed every two hours at the same time you do skin care. For an unconscious person, wipe the mouth with a gauze dipped in a rinsing solution or with a toothette.
- Use a non-alcohol based rinsing solution. Suggestions include:
  - baking soda (1 teaspoon) and water (2 cups)
  - salt (1/2 teaspoon), baking soda (1 teaspoon) and water (4 cups)
  - club soda
- Avoid over-the-counter mouthwashes that contain alcohol. The alcohol can make mouth tissues dry and increase the risk of infection.

IMPORTANT POINTS

- Because many bacteria grow in the mouth, wash your hands well before and after you give mouth care.
- Although toothettes are a convenient way to clean a person's mouth, they can break apart while in the mouth. Use them with caution.
- Do not give mouth care to a person who is lying flat as this may cause choking. For a person not able to raise the head, help to lie on the side and wipe any moisture remaining in the mouth with a gauze, clean cloth or toothette.
- If the person bites down on the toothbrush or toothette do not let go or try to yank it out. The jaw will eventually relax and you will be able to remove it then.
- Check in the person's mouth every day for signs of sores or other problems (see Mouth Problems, p.71).
- Do not put your fingers in the mouth of a person who is confused or sleepy. You run the risk of being bitten.
- Mouth care should be done at least twice a day.

POSITIONING SOMEONE IN BED

If someone is completely bedridden, is too weak to move, is paralysed or is unconscious, changing the position in bed will become one of your most important tasks. Long periods without moving can lead to pressure sores, which is a serious problem. Also, changing position helps keep the person's lungs free of mucus and can help ease pain.

How you can offer care

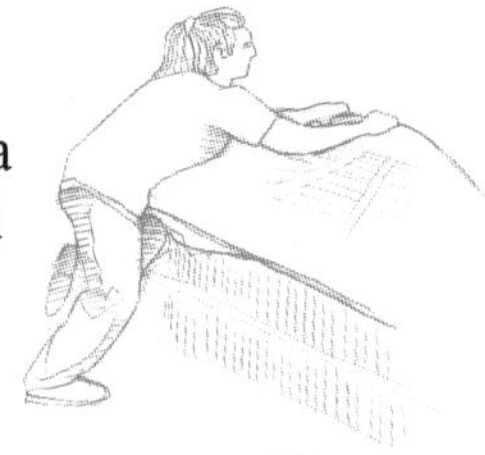

Often when a person finds a comfortable position, it is a strong temptation to stay without moving. You may need to insist when helping your loved one to shift in bed.

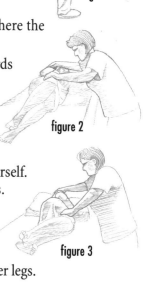

- Lower the head of the bed if this is possible.
- Loosen the bed covers and remove extra pillows.
- Move the person toward you on one side of the bed so after the turn the person will be in the centre of the bed. (See figure 1)

figure 1

- Use a turning sheet to help roll the person over (see Helping Someone Slide Up in Bed, p.34).
- If you do not have a turning sheet:
  - Stand on the opposite side of the bed from where the person is lying.
  - Place the person's far arm across the chest towards you. (See figure 2)

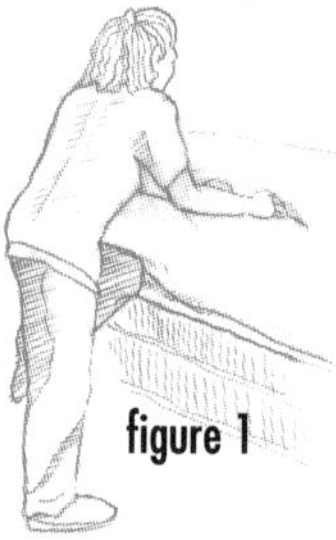

figure 2

  - Bend the far leg at the knee and bring the bent leg towards you. As you do this, the far shoulder will naturally start to move towards you. Place your hand behind the person's shoulder and roll the body toward yourself. Do not pull the person's arm while doing this. (See figure 3)
  - Place the person's knees and ankles together in a flexed position.

figure 3

- Place a flat pad or pillow under the knees and lower legs.

- Place a pillow lengthwise at the person's back and anchor it by pushing the edge under the person's back. Fold the outer side of the pillow under and tuck it in snugly against the person to give more support.
- Place a pillow lengthways under the person's thigh, bringing the leg forward so it does not rest on the lower leg. Position the leg comfortably.
- Place another pillow lengthways under the person's lower leg to prevent skin surfaces from rubbing together and to provide correct support. The pillow should extend well under the foot so the ankle and the foot do not drop and are kept level.
- Make sure the lower arm is in a comfortable position. The upper arm and hand may be more comfortable if they are placed on a pillow.
- When positioning someone on the back:
- Place two pillows lengthways at an angle. They should extend under the person's shoulders.

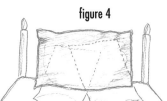

figure 4

- Place one pillow across the top of the two lengthways pillows so it is under the head and reaching to the shoulders. (See figure 4)
- A bar above the bed called a monkey or trapeze bar is a device that can help with moving in bed if the person has good upper body strength. Ask your home care nurse or occupational therapist.

ATTENTION TO PRESSURE AREAS

Skin breakdown or pressure sores can be a major source of discomfort for your loved one. Prevention of sores is a major part of physical care.

- Pressure sores usually happen over bony areas. (See figure 5)

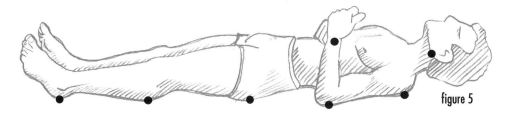

figure 5

- A back rub promotes blood supply to bony areas and can be relaxing as well.
- Encourage a person who can move unaided to change position in a bed or chair at least every two hours.
- Help a person who cannot move alone to turn every two hours during the day time and every four hours at night.

- Ask your home care nurse about using a mattress or cushions that prevent pressure.
- Check the person's skin for any reddened areas. These may turn into pressure sores.
- Massage the back and pressure areas with lotion after each turn. Use soft pressure and move your hands in a circular motion.
- Do this several times, using plenty of lotion so that the movement is smooth.
- Protect reddened areas with pillows, sheepskin, elbow and heel protectors. Ask your home care nurse about other protective devices such as special mattresses.
- Use pillows to support the person on a side lying position. The pillows can be gradually pulled back, so that after two hours the person will be on the back.
- Keep the skin clean and dry.
- Keep bed sheets dry and free of wrinkles.

HELPING SOMEONE SLIDE UP IN BED

As a person gets weaker it may be necessary to provide help to move in bed.

IMPORTANT POINTS

- Give pain medication about 30 minutes before turning if movement causes pain.
- Do not rub any reddened areas that remain red after you have changed the person's position. Tell your home care nurse about them.
- When helping a person to move, do not drag. Dragging causes friction which can cause skin to tear.
- Even if the person has discomfort when being turned, it is important to continue the turning routine.

How you can offer care

Someone who is lying in bed for long periods may need help to shift to a comfortable position, usually higher in the bed.

- Make sure the brakes are on, if the bed has wheels and lower the head of the bed.
- Raise the bed to about your waist level. If the bed cannot be raised, remember to use your knees not your back when lifting.
- Lower the side rail closest to you, if the bed has side rails.
- Check that no tubes or urine bags will be pulled with the move.
- Remove extra pillows and place a pillow against the headboard.

- Face the direction of the move. Your feet should be wide apart, toes pointing in the direction of the move. You can also place one knee on the bed to get close to the person. (See figure 6)
- Bend the person's knees.
- Place one hand under the person's back and the other hand under the thighs.
- Count to three and work together - the person pushes upwards and you lift toward the head of the bed.
- Do not pull the person's arms while you are helping with this positioning.

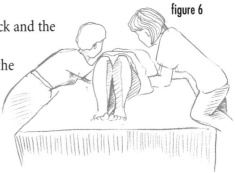

figure 6

Moving with a turning sheet

- Fold an extra sheet in half twice, to use as a turning sheet. Place the sheet under the person so it goes from mid-thigh to shoulder.
- Bend the person's knees.
- Stand beside the bed near the person's head, facing the feet.
- Grasp the turning sheet with one hand on each side of the person's shoulders.
- Count to three and work together - the person pushes upwards and you lift toward the head of the bed.

figure 7

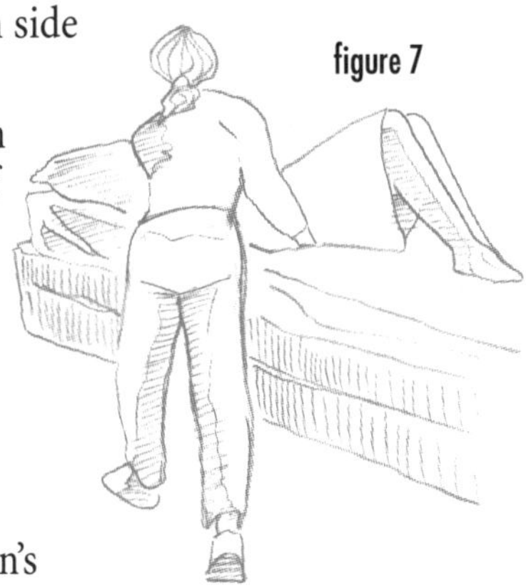

Moving with two people

- Both people face the direction of the move on opposite sides of the bed. (See figure 7)
- Bend the person's knees.
- Both people place their hands under the person's shoulder and waist.
- Count to three and work together - the person in bed pushes upwards and the other two lift toward the head of the bed.
- If a turning sheet is being used, grasp the sheet on each side, close to the person's shoulders and hips. On the count of three, the person pushes upwards and the other two lift toward the head of the bed. (See figure 8)

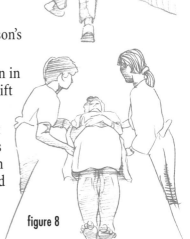

figure 8

MAKING A BED

For someone who is ill, the bed is often a place of refuge and comfort. If your loved one is confined to bed, the bedroom is the centre of activity and should be kept tidy and restful.

How you can offer comfort and care

It is important that the bed and surrounding area be kept clean to protect your loved one from problems such as infections. Change the sheets at least once a week and whenever they are soiled.

- Start by asking the person if this is a good time for you to change the bed. Wait for another time if tiredness seems to be a problem.
- Give a pain medication if needed, then wait about 30 minutes before you start.
- Collect the clean bedding and take it to the bedside. Place it on a nearby chair.
- Have a laundry basket close by so you can put soiled bedding directly into the basket.
- Ask the person if it is possible to sit in a chair for a few moments while you change the bed (see Moving Someone from Bed to Chair, p.40).
- Raise the bed to your waist level if this is possible. Lower the head of the bed so the bed is level.
- Remove the soiled bedding and place it in the laundry basket. Check that the mattress is dry and clean.
- Put a piece of plastic sheeting across the middle section of the mattress to protect it from moisture, if the person has diarrhea or is incontinent. An opened garbage bag or incontinence pad (plastic side down) under the bottom sheet will do.
- Be sure the sheets are flat and free of wrinkles to help prevent skin breakdown.
- Consider a turning sheet over the bottom sheet. This can protect the bottom sheet from becoming soiled and may save you changing the entire bed next time. A flannel sheet or light blanket folded in half will do as a draw sheet.
- Place the clean top sheet and blankets on the bed. When tucking in the top layers leave a little slack at the foot of the bed so the covers do not push down on the person's feet. If you are using a foot cradle, put it in place before you add the top layers.
- Replace the pillowcases daily or when soiled, tucking loose ends inside.

- If using incontinence pads, place a fresh one on the bottom sheet where the person's bottom will lie.
- Lower a hospital bed to average bed height when you are finished.
- Help the person back to bed.
- Remove garbage such as used tissues.

MAKING A BED WITH SOMEONE IN IT

When a person cannot get out of bed it is easier to have two people to change it.

- Collect your bedding and laundry basket. If using a hospital bed, raise the bed to waist level and lower the head so the bed is level.
- Remove the top sheets, blankets and all pillows except the one that remains under the person's head. Cover the person with a sheet for warmth and privacy.
- Loosen the bottom sheets all around the bed.
- Help the person to turn onto one side while giving support at the waist and shoulders. Make sure the head is resting on a pillow and the limbs are supported (see Positioning a Person in Bed, p.32).
- If there are two of you making the bed, one holds the person while the other rolls each layer of the bottom linens toward the centre of the bed, close to the person's back. If the person has been incontinent take this chance to do a wash, then cover the soiled linens with a towel.

figure 9

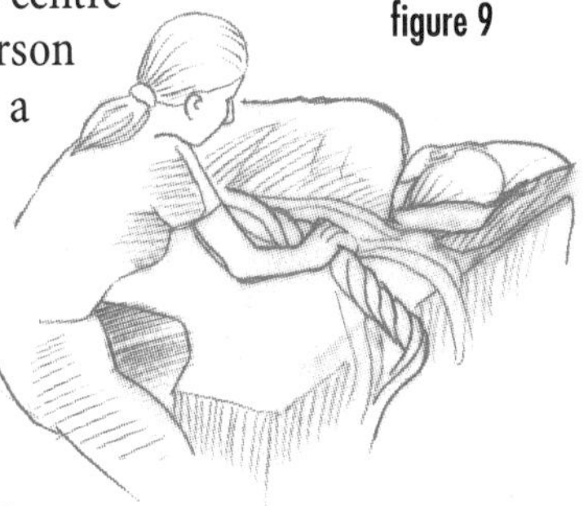

- If you are on your own, place a chair on the opposite side of the bed from you for the person to hang on to. If you have a hospital bed, raise the side rail and have the person hold on to that.
- Place the clean bottom sheet, rolled up lengthwise, against the rolled up dirty linens. Smooth out the flat half of the clean sheet and tuck it in. Repeat this process with each bottom layer of bedding you are using (mattress or foam, plastic sheeting, bottom sheet, draw sheet, turning sheet, incontinence pads). This will form a small hump. (See figure 9) 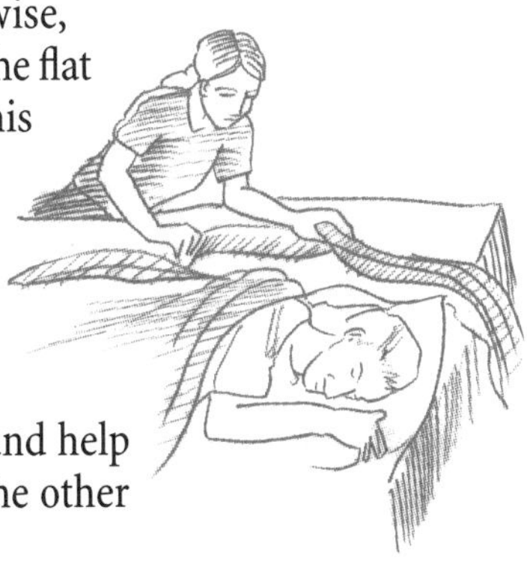
- Move the pillow to the other side of the bed and help the person turn over the rolls of bedding to the other side. Make sure to warn about the hump.

- If there are two of you, the other person now pulls through all the dirty linens and places them in the basket. Finish washing the person, then change the pyjamas. Pull through all layers of clean linen. Pull tightly to make the bottom layers straight and wrinkle free, then tuck in the sheets.

- If you are on your own, have another chair to hang on to, or raise the side rail, on the opposite side of the bed. Help the person roll over the hump. Go to the other side of the bed and do what a second person would have done.

- Help the person into a comfortable position. Replace the pillowcases and finish making the bed with a top sheet and blankets.

- Return the laundry basket and furniture to their regular places. Wash your hands.

HELPING WITH MOVING ABOUT

BODY MECHANICS (USING YOUR BODY CORRECTLY)

Body mechanics refers to the way you use your body during movement. It is especially important when you are doing something that can strain your joints. Paying attention to body mechanics during lifting or bending will help to prevent injury. A member of your health care team can show you how to do the movements safely.

What you need to know

The most important aspect of your own body mechanics is knowledge of your body's abilities. Pay attention to your own limitations. There are three terms you need to understand.

- Your centre of gravity is located at the middle of your body, about your hips.
- Your line of balance is an imaginary line, from head to foot, that divides your body into two equal parts.
- The base of support is the space between your feet that bears the weight of your body. (See figure 10)

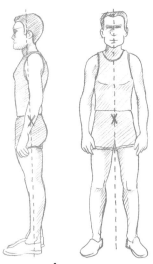

figure 10

- When moving or lifting a heavy object, reduce the strain on your back by keeping your line of balance close to your centre of gravity. Bend your knees instead of your back to keep you from leaning forward or backward.

- Open the distance between your feet to broaden your base of support. This distributes the extra weight you are bearing or lifting and decreases the strain on your back muscles.

- Get close to the object you are moving. Make sure your centre of gravity is as close to the object as possible.

- Use your arm and leg muscles, not your back, to do the work. When you are using your arms, keep the load close to your body. Also, your greatest lift power comes with pushing rather than pulling.

- Look at where you are and where you want to go. Think through the movement before you proceed.

LIFTING

When lifting a person, a few basic techniques done correctly can help prevent injury to everyone involved.

- Make sure obstacles or barriers are moved out of the way.

- Talk through the lift step by step so everyone involved understands the direction and purpose of the movement.

- Count to three before the movement begins, so everyone moves at the same time.

- Take a deep breath before you start and breathe regularly while lifting.

- Turn with your feet, pivot or step to avoid twisting your body.

- Always do the least amount of work to achieve your move. Have the person in bed help you as much as possible. Ask your home care nurse for advice about using a transfer belt.

IMPORTANT POINTS

- Do not attempt a lift that you think you cannot do alone. Two people are almost always better than one.
- If your back is weak or hurt do not attempt to lift or move someone.
- If you injure yourself, see your doctor right away.
- If the person begins to fall, do not resist the fall. Go with it gently and protect both of you from injury. Make sure to protect the person's head from hitting the floor.
- Once you reach the floor, take a few seconds to calm down and check that the person is all right.
- To help up from a fall, move the person to a chair first and then from the chair to the bed. Start with the person kneeling, then holding onto a chair and rising from there.

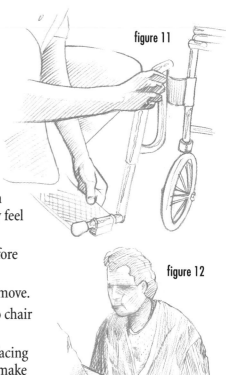

figure 11

MOVING SOMEONE FROM BED TO CHAIR

Getting out of bed can help lift someone's spirits and help to prevent bed sores.

How you can offer care

- Take your time. A person who has been lying in bed for any length of time may feel dizzy when sitting up.
- Make sure the dizziness has passed before making the move.
- Have all your equipment ready for the move.
- Put bed brakes on and lower the bed to chair height if that is possible.
- Place the chair at the head of the bed, facing the foot. If you are using a wheelchair, make sure the brakes are on and, when possible, remove the armrest and foot pedal closest to the bed. (See figure 11)
- Make sure you and the person both have on non-slip footwear.
- Raise the head of the bed as high as it will go.
- Move the person's legs over the side of the bed, then help the person slide forward to the edge of the bed. The feet should touch the floor or footstool. (See figure 12)
- Bend your knees and lean towards the person, keeping your back straight.
- Put the person's arms around your back, not around your neck. For someone too weak to grasp, place the arms over your shoulders with head resting on your shoulder. (See figure 13)
- Place your arms around the person's lower back or use the waist band, a turning sheet, towel or transfer belt around the back so you can support the person.

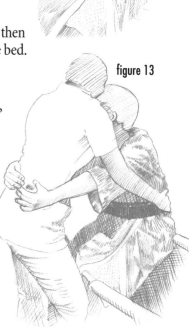

figure 12

figure 13

- Rock gently for momentum and count to three. In one continuous movement, stand, pivot, shuffle together backward until the chair touches the back of the knees, and lower the person into the chair. (See figures 14 and 15)
- Replace wheelchair armrest and foot pedal.

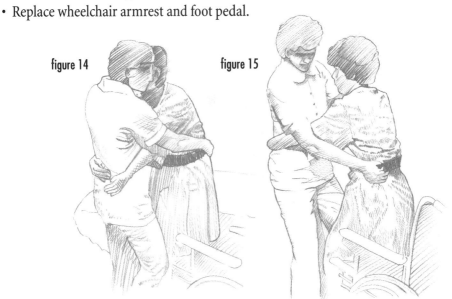

figure 14   figure 15

IMPORTANT POINTS

- If the person cannot stand, do not attempt this type of move. Ask your home care nurse about a mechanical lift or transfer aide.
- An occupational therapist or physiotherapist may be able to give you advice about how to help with moves. Ask about the use of a transfer belt.

WALKING

Although the person may be able to stand and walk, help may still be needed to prevent falls. Some people will be able to use a cane or walking device while others will need support.

How you can offer care

The most important thing for you to do is prevent your loved one from falling while walking.

- Move all obstacles from your path. Have a chair nearby in case the person needs a rest.
- Make sure both of you are wearing non-skid footwear.

- Provide your support on the person's weaker side. If a cane is used, have the person hold it on the stronger side. This will keep the weight on the side that can support it.
- Stand beside and slightly behind the person, facing the same direction. When necessary, remind the person to stand tall and to look ahead, not down at the floor.
- Put your arm around the person's waist and use your other hand to hold the person's elbow or hand. Stay close so that your entire body gives support. (See figure 16)
- Try using a belt or folded blanket around the person's waist so you can hang on to it to give added support.
- Ask a member of your health care team if a transfer belt or walker would make getting around any easier.

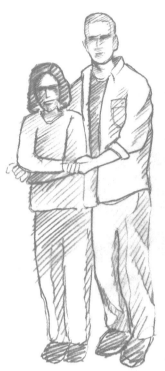

figure 16

IMPORTANT POINTS

- Ask an occupational therapist, physiotherapist or home care nurse for advice if you are unsure about helping a person with moving.
- Always remember the use of proper body mechanics.
- If the person begins to fall, do not resist the fall. Go with it gently and protect both of you from injury. Make sure to protect the person's head from hitting the floor.
- Once you reach the floor, take a few seconds to calm down and check that the person is all right.
- To help up from a fall, move the person to a chair first and then from the chair to the bed. Start with the person kneeling, then holding onto a chair and rising from there.
- **Call for help if:**
  - *you find the person on the floor and suspect an injury.*
  - *you cannot get the person off the floor.*
  - *you have doubts about moving the person by yourself.*

TOILETING

For some people, the need for help with toileting can be very embarrassing. This is particularly true for someone who is confined to bed.

What you need to know

- The person may need help to use the toilet, a commode, a urinal or a bedpan depending on mobility.
- When helping with toileting needs, respect your loved one's dignity.
- Be sensitive to the need for privacy.
- Be matter-of-fact about the activity to reduce embarrassment.

Bathroom

When the person is able to get up and go to the toilet, offer whatever help is needed. Stay close by.

- Make sure the bathroom floor is dry, the person has non-slip footwear and the path to the toilet is well-lit and free of obstacles.
- Place toilet paper within reach.
- Give privacy if the person can be left alone.
- Allow as much time as needed. The sound of running water might help someone who is having trouble urinating.
- Help with wiping-up as needed. Wipe from front to back.
- Help the person to wash when finished, then wash your own hands.
- Take your time getting back to the bed or chair.

Commodes

Commodes are portable toilets in the shape of a chair. They can be positioned close to the bed of a person who is able to get up but too weak to walk to a bathroom.

- Be sure the brakes are locked on the commode.
- Use the techniques described in Moving from Bed to Chair (p.40) to help the person move to, and use the commode.
- Let the person do as much as possible. Have toilet paper within reach.
- Help the person to wash hands.
- Empty the commode bucket as soon as you have helped the person back to the bed or chair.
- Wash your hands and return the commode to its usual place.

Urinals

Urinals are small collection bottles that men can use for passing urine. They come in different shapes and sizes and are usually made of plastic. Some are made of metal or moulded cardboard.

- Some men are able to use the urinal lying down, while others prefer sitting on the edge of the bed or standing up. If the person wants to stand, offer support.
- If the person uses the urinal in bed, raise the head of the bed for comfort. Make sure the foot of the bed is down so that urine does not spill out.
- Keep the urinal emptied and thoroughly rinsed after every use. This will help to prevent spills and offensive odours. If you rinse with cold water and baking soda, it will keep odour down.
- Wash your hands after emptying the urinal.
- If the person wants help using the urinal, be sure the penis is placed directly into the urinal and that the urinal is tilted downward.

Bedpans

Most people find a bedpan uncomfortable and awkward to use but if a person is not able to get out of bed, it may be necessary.

- Warm up a bedpan if you want to by rinsing it with hot water and then drying.
- Try some talcum powder on top of the bedpan so it does not stick to the skin.
- Place the bedpan by asking a person who is strong enough to lie with knees bent and feet flat on the mattress. Help lift the person's bottom while you slide the bedpan under.

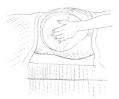

- Alternatively, help the person roll away from you. Place an incontinence pad on the mattress, put the bedpan on the mattress where the person's bottom will be and help the person roll back onto the pan. (See figures 17, 18 and 19)

figure 17

- Raise the head of the bed to increase comfort. Have the foot of the bed down so that urine will not pour out by mistake.

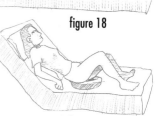

- Make sure the person is wiped clean and dry.

figure 18

- Cover the bedpan before removing it to prevent spilling. Empty it in the toilet and clean. Rinse with cold water and baking soda to keep it odour free.
- Wash your hands and help the person to wash.

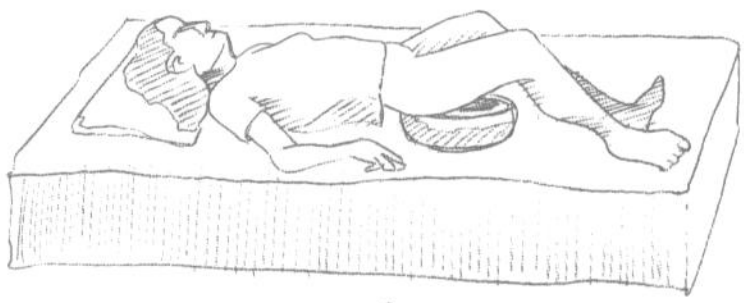

figure 19

FOOD AND FLUID NEEDS

DECREASING APPETITE

What you can expect

Enjoying food and drink together is a part of our culture. It is difficult to watch someone you love eat less than usual.

- A decreasing appetite is normal because the body cannot digest food as it once did.
- The person may refuse solids and will only drink liquids.
- There may be a noticeable weight loss. This may happen because of the disease, no matter how much is eaten.
- A changing sense of taste may alter the enjoyment of food. Sometimes this is only temporary.
- Bitter tastes may develop or sometimes food may seem too sweet.
- Some people develop distaste for meat or for certain textures of foods and certain smells.

How you can offer comfort and care

Try to find ways to tempt the person's appetite and give nourishing foods but remember that there is no harm going without food sometimes. The important thing is that the person continue to drink fluids (see Preventing Dehydration, p.51).

- Try new spices and flavourings for foods. It is common for a person's preferences to change during illness.
- Avoid highly seasoned or salty foods.
- Add sauces and gravies to dry food.
- Flavour food with sugar, basil, seasonings, lemon juice or mint.
- Add fruit and juice to milkshakes, custards, ice cream and puddings.
- Marinate meat in soya sauce, sweet juices or sweet wines.
- Try alternative high protein foods such as eggs, poultry or fish for someone who has developed a dislike of meat.
- Give high protein, high calorie snacks such as eggnogs, cream soups and ice-cream.

- Choose foods that are soft and easy to eat.
- Avoid foods that have similar textures to the foods the person dislikes.
- Try serving water, tea or soft drinks to take a strange taste away. Sometimes citrus juices such as lemon added to foods can make a taste more normal.
- Increase or decrease the sweetness of foods if the person finds this improves flavours.
- Vary food colour and use garnishes to make food attractive.
- Choose the person's favourite foods, served in small portions five or six times a day.
- Offer small, frequent meals at times when the person has least pain and is well rested.
- Have dentures relined or try a product such as Polygrip™ if they are loose.
- Tell your home care nurse if nausea is a problem. Medications that stop nausea can be very helpful.
- Encourage the person to exercise, if possible, to encourage appetite. Even simple exercises such as leg lifts done in bed can help.
- Make breakfast a nourishing meal as appetite tends to decrease as the day progresses.
- Try a glass of beer or wine to stimulate the appetite unless this is not recommended by the doctor.
- Encourage the person to eat food low in fat, chew slowly and pause occasionally during the meal to avoid feeling full too quickly.
- Freshen and clean the person's mouth before and after eating.
- Make meal time a social occasion. A person who is not able to go to the table will enjoy having you sit at the bedside and perhaps have a meal there.
- Eat in a calm and relaxed atmosphere.
- Serve food on small dishes so the amount does not look like so much.
- Offer cold plates such as cottage cheese and fruit plates if the smell of food is a problem.
- Try nutritional supplements such as Ensure™ or Boost™. New flavours are being developed all the time. Even if the person does not like the taste of one supplement, it is worth checking regularly for new ones. Also, to improve the taste they can be frozen and eaten like ice cream or thickened to make them into a pudding.

NUTRITIONAL SUPPLEMENTS

Food supplements (commercial or home-made) can help people who are losing weight or having difficulty chewing or swallowing. These drinks or puddings provide an easy and convenient source of calories and protein.

Commercial food supplements

Many commercially prepared supplements can be purchased at your local pharmacy or grocery stores. These include supplements for people who are unable to tolerate lactose or sugar. As well as some of the brand names indicated below, there are generic brands that may cost less. Several of the products are also available with fibre added. Diabetics should not use a product that contains any of the types of sugar. If you are not sure about sugar types, ask your dietitian or home care nurse.

Contain lactose	Do not contain lactose	Contain sugar only
Carnation Instant Breakfast™	Resource Fruit Beverage™	Caloreen™
Meritene™ - liquid - powder	Ensure™	Polycose™
Sustacal™ - liquid - pudding	Ensure Plus™	
	Ensure Fruitango™	
	Sustain™ Attain™	
	Nutrisure™ (Ensure Pudding)	
	Boost™ and Boost Plus™	

Home-made food supplements

Commercial nutritional supplements are loaded with nutrients but some people do not like the taste.

- Try offering a powershake or power-slushie instead.
  - A powershake is a milkshake with added nutritional powders that you can buy in pharmacies and health food stores. It is a meal in a glass. You can make the shake in a blender with milk, ice cream and the nutritional powder. Lactose-free products such as LactaidTM or Rice Dream™ (a non-dairy cream) can also be used. Flavour as the person wishes.
  - Power-slushies can be used when the person is producing a lot of mucus and you want to avoid dairy products. In a blender, mix the nutritional powder with crushed ice and fruit juice.

• Other recipes you might try provide similar calories and protein to the commercial supplements. Some examples are:

High protein milk *(180 calories, 15 grams protein)*
Blend   1 cup milk (250 mL)
1/4 cup skim milk powder (50 mL)

Milkshake *(380 calories, 20 grams protein)*
Blend   1 cup high protein milk (250 mL)
3/4 cup ice cream (200 mL)

Peanut Butter Shake *(510 calories, 20 grams protein)*
Blend   3/4 cup ice cream (200 mL)
1/2 cup milk (125 mL)
1/4 cup skim milk powder (50 mL)
2 Tbsp. peanut butter (30 mL)

Strawberry Delight *(765 calories, 20 grams protein)*
Blend   1 cup ice cream (250 mL)
3/4 cup milk (200 mL)
3/4 cup half and half cream (200 mL)
1/4 cup skim milk powder (50 mL)
2 Tbsp. strawberry jam (30 mL)

Yogurt Shake *(290 calories, 15 grams protein)*
Blend   3/4 cup plain yogurt (200 mL)
1/4 cup skim milk powder (50 mL)
1/2 cup apple juice (125 mL)
1 Tbsp. sugar or honey (15 mL)

Super Pudding *(1,065 calories, 35 grams protein)*
Blend   1 pkg. (41/2 oz., 113 grams) instant pudding
2 cups milk (500 mL)
2 Tbsp. oil (30 mL)
3/4 cup skim milk powder (200 mL)

Soup Plus *(295 calories, 20 grams protein)*

Blend   1 cup cream soup (250 mL)

         2 oz. cooked meat or poultry (50 grams)

         2 Tbsp. skim milk powder (50 mL)

Fruit Shake *(350 calories)*

Blend   1/2 cup whole milk

         1/2 cup canned peaches or other fruits

         1 cup vanilla ice cream

LIQUID FEEDINGS

These recipes can be useful if the person has problems swallowing or chewing food.

Hot Blender (Yield: 6 - 6 oz. servings, 155 calories per serving)

| Blend until smooth and heat | 1 cup cooked meat (chopped fine) or canned baby food meat
1 cup cooked carrots or other vegetables
and heat 2 small cooked potatoes
2 cups whole milk
1 cup canned or home-made cream soup |

Cold Blender (Yield: 6 - 6 oz. servings, 265 calories per serving)

| Blend and add syrup or flavour if desired | 2 cups ice cream and add
2 1/2 cups whole milk
1 cup cereal cream
1/2 cup sugar |

IMPORTANT POINTS

- For the safe use of home-made supplements:
  - keep refrigerated and discard after 24 hours.
  - do not keep at room temperature for longer than two hours.
- Follow these instructions carefully as these supplements spoil easily.

GIVING HELP WITH EATING

The act of eating can cause problems. As well as having no appetite the person may not have the energy to eat.

How you can offer comfort and care

Even though your loved one may be having difficulty eating, there are some things you can do to make it easier.

- Encourage the person to rest after meals, but keep the head of the bed elevated to help digestion.
- Make adjustments to the diet if the person can no longer wear dentures. Soft foods or small bite-size portions of meat, softened with gravy are ideal.
- Remember that the person may forget to eat. Offer small snacks throughout the day rather than waiting to be asked.
- Assess the person's ability to chew and swallow before you serve solid foods. For someone who can swallow but cannot chew, a puree or pudding would be most effective. For someone who can chew, keep food pieces small so less energy is needed to eat.
- Give finger foods if the person prefers or can only eat with fingers. This will help to maintain a level of independence.
- Be sure that the person's head is well supported and upright when eating or being fed.
- Use bibs or large napkins when necessary to help keep clothing and bedding clean.
- Use a spoon instead of a fork when you are feeding someone. This will prevent accidental stabs with a fork prong. Also, a long-handled spoon will help you place the food far enough into the mouth.
- Offer small spoonfuls and place food at the front of the mouth. Wait until the last spoonful is swallowed before offering the next.
- Give liquids and solids separately.
- Practice feeding with a friend or family member. Switch roles so you are aware of both sides of the feeding experience.
- Keep a small kidney basin or bowl close by. Nausea and vomiting can happen very suddenly so be prepared.

IMPORTANT POINTS

- Ask your pharmacist or home care nurse about medications that may improve appetite.
- Tell your home care nurse if nausea, dry or sore mouth, or problems swallowing are affecting the person's appetite.
- Never force someone to eat or drink.
- If the person coughs or chokes frequently when eating or drinking, stop. Ask your home care nurse if it is safe to continue feeding.

PREVENTING DEHYDRATION

Fluids provide the body with nutrition, help to flush out body waste products and help keep cells and skin healthy. If your loved one is no longer able to drink enough fluids, dehydration may occur, meaning there is not enough fluid in the body tissues. Dehydration can cause weakness, nausea, confusion and restlessness.

What you need to know

- One of the first indications of dehydration is less urine being produced.
- In dehydration, the colour of the urine will be very dark yellow or tea-coloured with a strong odour.
- Wastes will not be removed from the body and the person may become confused.

IMPORTANT POINTS

- As the person grows weaker it is more important to drink than eat.
- Aim for about two litres or eight to 10 glasses of fluid a day.
- If dehydration happens because the person is not drinking, giving fluids by placing a needle under the skin may be an alternative (see Hypodermoclysis, p.52).

How you can offer comfort and care

- Always have fluids close at hand. These include water, juice, coffee, tea, ice chips, broths and nutritional supplements. Water flavoured with lemon juice is refreshing.
- Change the fluids often to keep them fresh.
- Use ice chips or popsicles as excellent ways to give fluids. Also, they help to keep the mouth moist and feeling fresh.
- Raise the person's head when helping to drink. Use a couple of pillows or gently support the base of the head with your hand. It is almost impossible to drink when lying flat.
- Ask the person to take small sips and not big gulps to help prevent choking.
- Use a straw that bends when the person is strong enough to suck on it.
- Try a spill-free thermos bottle or cup to make drinking easier if lips no longer fit tightly around the rim of a glass.
- Use a gentle reminder if the person forgets to swallow. Sometimes softly stroking the side of the throat will help to stimulate swallowing.
- Offer fluids that are somewhat thick and easier to swallow such as milkshakes and applesauce, if the person has difficulty swallowing.

HYPODERMOCLYSIS

If your loved one cannot take enough fluids by mouth and it is thought that more fluids might improve the person's quality of life, the doctor may decide to do a procedure called hypodermoclysis.

What you need to know

figure 20

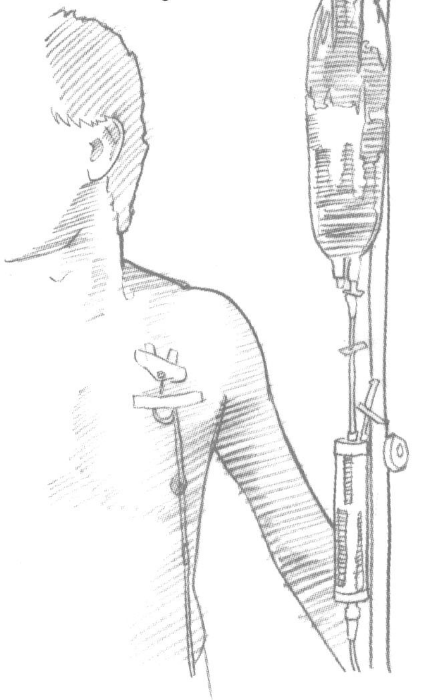

Hypodermoclysis means giving fluid into body tissues by a small needle placed just under the skin (subcutaneous). The needle is attached to a plastic tube and a bag of water. An intravenous is seldom used to give a person more fluids because the subcutaneous method is easier, safer, and restricts the person's movement less. (See figure 20)

- The insertion of the needle is the same as described for subcutaneous medications (see p.59).
- The home care nurse will start the treatment, and will help with maintaining it. (If you are taught how to start the treatment, see Starting a Hypodermoclysis p.144 to remind yourself of the procedure.)
- The fluid can be given throughout the day and night or may be given at night when the person is sleeping.
- The location of the needle may not need to be changed for up to seven days.
- Medications may be given through this needle.
- The needle is very small. It may sting when first inserted but should not cause any further pain.
- Fluid may collect under the skin at the location of the needle but it will gradually be absorbed into the body.

How can you offer comfort and care

Reassure the person that this procedure is:
- a comfort measure.
- a safe method of giving fluid.
- easy to turn off when sitting up or walking.

For and against hypodermoclysis

There is a debate about whether or not a person who is dying should be given fluids by hypodermoclysis. You may be asked for your opinion on this. The following are the arguments for and against this treatment.

For the treatment

- Poor fluid intake causes dehydration and can lead to confusion, hallucinations, restlessness and nausea. Dehydration should be avoided because:
  - if the person is on opioids, there is a greater risk of toxicity from them (see Opioid Toxicity, p.96).
  - the person is at increased risk for bedsores and constipation.
  - dry mouth and thirst is a concern.

Against the treatment

- When the person is dehydrated there may be less awareness of pain and distress.
- Dehydration results in reduced respiratory and gastric fluids, urinary output, and swelling, all of which may be more comfortable for the person.

Remember that each person and situation is different. A decision whether or not to start hypodermoclysis can only be made by your loved one, you and the health care team planning together.

MEDICATIONS

Your attention to the proper care and use of medications will help increase the benefits they offer.

What you need to know

Your loved one may have many medications prescribed and it is essential that these be handled carefully and accurately. If the person is not able to do this alone, you can help in several ways.

- Keeping records of medications is very important, especially when regular doses of pain relief are being given. A good recording system will help you keep organized.
- A chart showing a list of medications, when they are taken, and the dose will help the doctor know if there is a need to change the drug or the dose. (See Home Medication Schedule, Appendix III, p.135).
- Heat and light can change the chemical composition of some medicines.
- Most medications are best stored in a cool, dark place.
- Some medications need to be kept in the refrigerator. Make sure they will not freeze and that children cannot get at them.

IMPORTANT POINTS ABOUT ANY METHOD OF GIVING MEDICATION

- Never try to give oral medications to someone asleep or unconscious.
- Use the right medicine, in the right amount, at the right time.
- Administer the medication by the correct method - liquids, tablets, drops, ointment, sprays, suppositories, injections.
- If medications are ordered by more than one doctor or are over-the-counter products, ask your doctor or pharmacist if they are all safe to take together.
- Check with your home care nurse or pharmacist if you notice sudden behaviour changes, hallucinations or other mild or severe reactions.
- Keep medications out of the reach of a person who is confused.
- If the person is using products from a health food store, or over-the-counter remedies, tell your doctor or pharmacist so you avoid the risk of conflicts. For example, some herbs may interfere with prescribed medications.
- **Call for help if:**
  - *the needle site becomes red, swollen, leaks, bleeds or causes discomfort.*

- Many medications have an expiry date. If a drug is too old to use, talk to your home care nurse about proper disposal of it.
- Medications should be kept in a safe place out of the reach of children or anyone who might take them accidentally.

• Do not talk in public about the medications you have in your home and keep them in a secure place out of sight. There is always a risk of someone trying to break in to steal them.

How you can offer care

Follow the instructions for proper use of medications and do not hesitate to ask for advice if you are not sure.

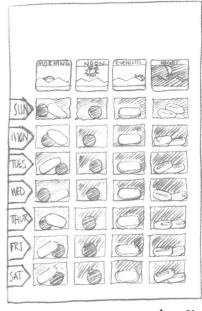

figure 21

• Discuss with your home care nurse and pharmacist how you can set up a schedule for the medications and how you can help the person take the medications properly.

• Try to use the same pharmacist all the time. That person will understand your situation and be in a better position to answer your questions.

• Remember that it might take a few days to get a new supply of a prescription drug.

  • Keep track of how much you have left of any medication and how long it will last.

  • Keep all your stock of medication in one place.

  • Have someone in charge of keeping track of what is needed. Be sure to order more before the present supply runs out.

• It is very easy to mix up medications, especially when several different ones are being used.

  • Try to organize the way you store drugs so it is easy to tell them apart.

  • Keep a medication chart nearby for quick checking.

  • Try colour coding - mark each label with a coloured dot, then put a matching dot beside the medication's name on a chart. This will help you be sure you are giving the right one.

  • Check each medication twice as you are preparing it. Read the label when you pick up the container and again when you are finished preparation to be sure it is the correct one.

  • Ask your pharmacist or home care nurse about a medication dispenser to help organize a long list of drugs to be taken. These dispensers are called dosettes. Your pharmacist may also be able to help organize the medications into groupings contained in packaging called blister or bubble packs. (See figure 21)

- When you get a prescription filled, ask about side effects so you know what to expect. Be sure the medication is safe with other drugs being used. (Have a list with you of other medications being used.)
- Find out if there is any food or drink (such as alcohol) that might interfere with the benefits of the drug.

GIVING MEDICATIONS BY MOUTH

Medications given by mouth are also called oral medications. They include anything that is swallowed - pills, capsules, tablets, lozenges, syrups and elixirs. Oral medications are the safest and easiest way to get a medication into the body.

- Wash your hands before you handle the medication.
- Most oral medications are meant to be swallowed right away.
- Some oral medications such as lozenges are sucked or chewed. Lozenges should not be swallowed whole.
- For pills, capsules or tablets, offer a glass of water or juice to help the person swallow. Suggest a sip of fluid before taking the pill to lubricate the mouth and help swallowing. Avoid milk unless you have been told the medication should be taken this way.
- Help the person sit up or raise the head to make swallowing easier. Never give an oral medication to someone who is lying down as this could lead to choking.
- Some medicines are hard on the stomach. Do not give oral medications on an empty stomach unless that is what the instructions say to do. Check the labels on the package or bottle and do what they say.
- Be sure a medication has been swallowed before you record it on the medication chart.
- If the person is having trouble swallowing pills, try some of these tips.
  - Offer some water first to moisten the throat, place pills at the back of the tongue and follow with more water. Try to encourage the person to relax the throat while swallowing.
  - Mix pills in applesauce, jam, ice cream, sherbet or pudding - anything that has substance enough to carry the pills down the throat.
  - Some pills can be crushed and then mixed but check first with your doctor or pharmacist which ones can be crushed.
  - Small pills can be put into a gelatin capsule by your pharmacist, then swallowed together in one capsule instead of separately.
- Ask your pharmacist if the medication comes in a liquid form. If so, talk to your doctor about changing the prescription.

- If the person is taking a liquid medication and does not like the taste, keep the bottle in the refrigerator or disguise the taste with another liquid like pop, juice or milk. Use different liquids so the bad taste will not become associated with any one drink.
- If the person is still not able to swallow the medications, ask your pharmacist or doctor about alternative methods such as a suppository or skin patch. It is important that the medication schedule not be interrupted.
- If the person is having side effects or the medication is not working the way you expect it to, talk with your home care nurse.

GIVING MEDICATIONS BY SUPPOSITORIES

A suppository is a medication moulded into a small solid shape that can be put into the rectum. This route is a useful alternative when medications cannot be given by mouth. Suppositories are used most often to relieve pain, constipation, nausea, vomiting or fever.

- Most suppositories are kept in the refrigerator but do not use one directly from there. It will be cold and could be uncomfortable. Let it warm up first.
- To give a suppository, you will need latex gloves and some lubricant such as K-Y Jelly™. Collect everything you need.
- Help the person into a position that will make it easy to insert the suppository. The best position is lying on the left side, with the upper leg bent forward.
- Put on the glove and lubricate the suppository (if you do not have a lubricant, wetting the suppository will make it easier to insert).
- Ask the person to take a deep breath and try to relax the muscles around the anus. Slow, rhythmic deep breathing will help to relax muscles.
- Spread the buttocks with one hand to expose the anus. Then, with the other hand, slide the suppository inside about two inches.
- The suppository may trigger the urge to have a bowel movement but encourage the person to hold on. The suppository needs 10 to 15 minutes to dissolve.

GIVING MEDICATIONS ABSORBED THROUGH THE SKIN (TRANSDERMAL)

Some medications are absorbed through the skin. Most of these come in creams or ointments that are put on the skin. Some come in patches that are put on the skin and taped in place, or have their own adhesive.

- For creams and ointments it may be important to wear gloves so that you do not come into contact with the medication. Ask your pharmacist.
- When putting on medication patches:
    - select a clean, dry area of skin on the front or back, above the waist. (The medication is absorbed best at this location). Do not apply the patch to oily, broken, burned, cut or irritated skin. To clean the skin area, use only clear water - no soap or alcohol. Be sure that the area is completely dry before applying the patch.
    - clip a hairy area with scissors but do not shave it.
    - remove the skin patch from its protective pouch and peel off the strip. Try not to touch the sticky side.
    - put the sticky side against the skin.
    - press the patch firmly for about 10 to 20 seconds with the palm of your hand. Be sure that the edges stick to the person's skin.

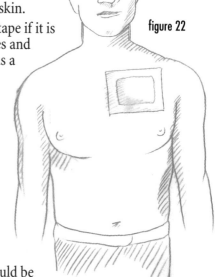

figure 22

    - tape the patch in place with paper tape if it is not self-adhesive. Tape the top, sides and bottom so the patch looks like it has a frame around it. (See figure 22)
    - wash your hands.

- Apply each new patch to a different skin area to avoid irritation. Remove the old patch before applying another one.
- Replace the patch with a new one in a different area if it comes off accidentally or the skin under the patch becomes irritated. Be sure the new skin area is clean and dry.
- Write a schedule of when patches should be changed. Some people write a date directly onto the patch. It is easy to lose track.
- Dispose of used and leftover unused patches immediately. The procedure for disposal varies across the province so ask your home care nurse how it is done in your community.

GIVING SUBCUTANEOUS MEDICATIONS

Subcutaneous means 'just under the skin.' For a subcutaneous injection, a tiny needle is placed under the skin (subcutaneous tissue). This needle is left in place and taped securely for repeated use.

Most medications for controlling symptoms can be given by subcutaneous injections rather than by intravenous (IV). The subcutaneous method is easier, safer and does not restrict the person's movement as an IV would. In some case an IV is needed if the person needs IV antibiotics or blood products but this is seldom necessary to keep a person comfortable.

What you need to know

If your loved one is not able to take medications by mouth, a subcutaneous injection may be used.

figure 23

- If you want to learn how to start a subcutaneous needle, the home care nurse will teach you (see Inserting and Removing a Subcutaneous Needle, Appendix VI, p.138).
- Whether or not you choose to insert the subcutaneous needle, the home care nurse will start and will help maintain this treatment.
- The needle is very small. It may sting when first inserted but should not cause any further pain.
- The needle is put into the abdomen or chest usually but can also be put into the thigh, upper arm or back.
- The needle has a tube. A rubber stopper can be attached to the tube through which medication is given. (See figure 23)
- Your home care nurse may pre-load medication into a syringe and ask you to give it because of the time or frequency of the dose. This may mean giving the medication at scheduled times or when requested by the person.
- Your home care nurse will show you how to wipe the rubber stopper with an alcohol swab and inject the medication.

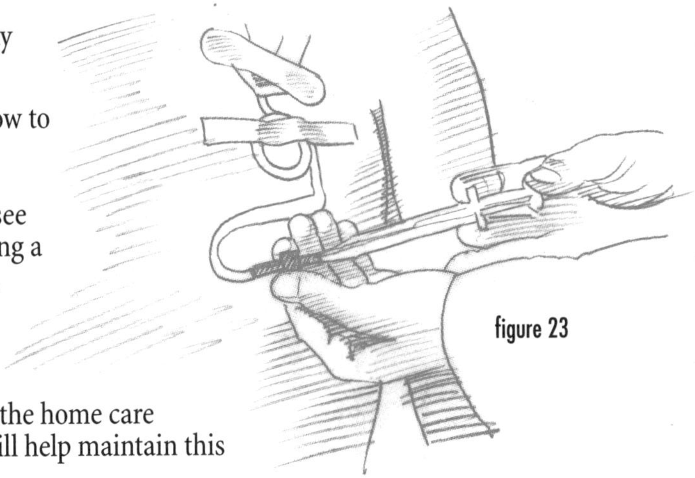

- Another way of giving medications is by attaching a pump that will include a small container of medication. There are different types of pumps. The person may be able to self-administer the medication using a pump such as an Edmonton injector, or there are computerized pumps that can be set to administer the medication continuously. (See figures 24 and 25)

- Sometimes the pump is provided through the hospital or you may need to rent it. Your home care nurse can help you organize this.

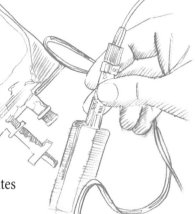

figure 24

- A subcutaneous needle is usually left in place between four to seven days depending on the type of medication going into it. However, some sites have been known to last for 30 days or more.

How you can offer comfort

- Explain the reason for the subcutaneous needle by saying that it is important that medications continue to be given even when swallowing is difficult.

- Reassure the person that once the needle is inserted there should be no further discomfort.

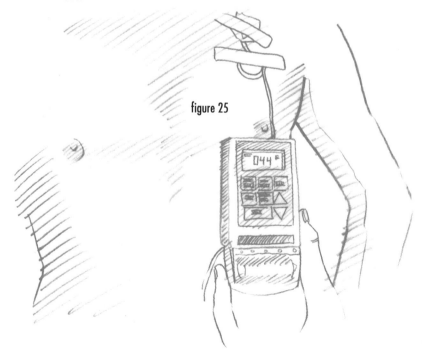

figure 25

Care of Physical Problems

PAIN

ASSESSING THE PAIN

When someone complains of pain, it is usually at a particular location in the body. However, a general feeling of not being well is sometimes experienced and described as pain.

What you need to know

To help the person it is important to assess the pain. It is also important to know that people express pain in different ways.

- Assessing pain is an ongoing process. You need to know as much as you can about the person's pain at any given time.
- The feeling of pain may be worse if the person is having other physical symptoms such as nausea. Also, worry, fear, boredom and loneliness may make the experience of pain worse. It is better to attend to these particular needs than to increase pain medications.
- Understanding more about the pain will help you to provide comfort and will let you know if the help you are giving is working.

How you can offer comfort and care

No one is more expert about the pain than the person who is feeling it. If the person you are caring for complains of pain, believe it. Even if there is no complaint, ask about any signs of discomfort you see.

- The experience of pain is different for each person. By asking the following questions, you will be able to provide the doctor or home care nurse with information that can help control the pain.
  - Where is the pain? Is it one particular place or is it all over? Ask "Can you point to where the pain is? Is it deep inside or on the surface? Is there more than one type of pain?"
  - When did the pain begin - an hour ago, yesterday, months ago?
  - How often does the pain occur?
  - How long does the pain last - minutes, hours? Does it come and go, or is it constant?
  - What does the pain feel like? Ask the person to describe it. Provide examples of words to use - stabbing, burning, aching, throbbing, piercing.
  - How much does it hurt? It is helpful to ask the person to rate the pain on a scale from zero to 10, where zero is no pain and 10 is the worst yet.

- What could have started the pain - was it movement, eating, pressure, the way the person was lying or sitting?
- What makes the pain go away - rest, massage, movement?
- To what degree is the pain limiting normal activities?
- What other symptoms are present?

- The ongoing use of a pain rating scale can give valuable information on the person's pain experience over time. A rating scale used everyday can help evaluate the pain. This information can be put on a graph. From the graphed results, your home care nurse can help you decide if you should contact the doctor for a change of medication. (See Symptom Assessment Scale, Appendix IV, p.136 and Wong-Baker Pain Rating Scale, below).

> **IMPORTANT POINTS**
>
> - **Call for help if:**
>   - *a new pain occurs - not the one the person usually has.*
>   - *pain continues after you have given three break through doses in 24 hours (see information on 'break through' in next section Managing Pain with Medications).*
>   - *there is a rapid increase in the intensity of the pain.*
>   - *there is sudden acute pain.*
>   - *you notice sudden confusion (see Confusion, p.86).*

| 0 | 2 | 4 | 6 | 8 | 10 |

MANAGING PAIN WITH MEDICATIONS

Someone who has constant pain needs regular pain medication to control it.

What you need to know

- The goal of pain management is to keep someone alert with the pain under control. It takes time and experimentation to arrive at the exact combination of medications that will keep a person feeling this way. You can shorten this process by recording positive or negative effects of a new medication and talking to the doctor about the results.
- A record of the pain and of regular scheduled pain medication and break through doses will help the doctor adjust the dose (see Assessing the Pain, p.62).
- Medications that provide relief from pain are called analgesics. Two basic groups of analgesics are opioids and non-opioids. (See World Health Organization Analgesic Ladder, p.64.)

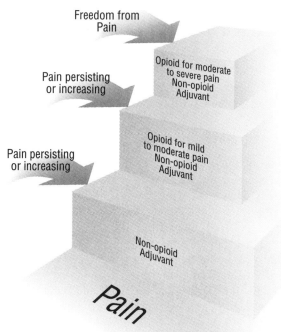

World Health Organization Analgesic Ladder

- Opioids are analgesics defined by the Canadian Narcotic Control Act as controlled substances. (Although the word narcotic is often used for these medications, the proper word is opioid.) They are used for moderate to severe pain.
- Non-opioids are probably the most commonly used medications and they include products to ease pain and to lower fever. They are prescribed usually for mild to moderate pain.

How you can offer comfort and care

Some basic guidelines apply to the use of any pain relief medication.

- Give the medication on schedule even if there is no pain at the time so the pain stays away. Once the pain returns, it becomes more difficult to control. (There is a four-hour timer available that can help you keep track of the schedule for pain medication. If this would be helpful to you, ask your pharmacist.)
- Plan to give your care just after a medication has taken effect to reduce discomfort. Most pain medications will take effect within 30 minutes. This is useful to know if you have to change a dressing or move a person around in bed.
- Pain medication, when taken regularly, is just as effective taken by mouth as by any other route. Only when the person cannot take pills by mouth are alternative routes such as injections or suppositories considered.

Things to remember about opioid pain medicines

- Short-acting opioids require a dose every three to four hours to keep the person completely comfortable. Set an alarm to wake yourself up for night time doses. Otherwise the person will wake up in pain.

- Keep track of pain relief. If the person has been on a stable dose of pain medication for three to four days, the doctor can prescribe a longer acting opioid. Some of these last 12 hours or 24 hours, and one is available in a patch that lasts for three days. The person's pain must be under control for these to work well.

- Sometimes pain will 'break through' even when it should be controlled by medication. For example, a person may feel mild or even severe pain two hours before the next scheduled dose. When this happens, a 'break through' dose of the pain medication is often ordered. Break through medication can be given every hour if necessary to a maximum of three times in 24 hours. If the person has needed more than this to control the pain, tell your doctor. Keep track of every break through medication the person takes to help the doctor adjust the regular dose. (See Home Break Through chart, Appendix V, p.137).

- Remember that opioids are potent medications and should be kept safely out of sight and out of reach of children and others. As with any other medication, do not talk in public about the fact that you have these drugs in your home. Otherwise there is a risk someone may try to steal them.

- Have at least a one-week supply of opioid medications on hand.

- Ask your home care nurse how you should dispose of unused opioids.

Things to remember about non-opioid pain medications

There are some steps you can take to help make pain relief more effective and reduce unwanted effects.

- Unless you are told otherwise, offer the medication with food to lessen stomach upset.

- Acetaminophen (Tylenol™) can be taken on an empty stomach to improve the way it is absorbed.

- Watch for signs of bleeding or bruising as some of these medications can affect the blood's clotting.

- Watch for signs of decreased urine output.

SIDE EFFECTS OF OPIOIDS

Drowsiness

When a medication is given for the first time, it can have an effect on the nervous system.

- The person may become sleepy. This may clear up in a few days or last as long as a week. Remember that the person may also be tired from exhaustion and lack of sleep.
- Let the person cat nap whenever desired. Just be sure you are able to rouse the person unless so seriously ill that this is not possible.

Nausea and vomiting

When first used, strong opioids can cause queasiness or even make a person throw up. These problems usually disappear in a few days.

- Nausea and vomiting can also be an effect of other medications the person is taking or a result of the illness itself.
- Encourage resting in bed for the first hour or so after taking pain medication.
- Remind the person that pain can cause nausea and vomiting, and if this is the case, the medication may help relieve it.
- Ask the doctor about an anti-nausea medication to be taken for three or four days when starting a new opioid or having a dose increase (see Nausea and Vomiting, p.81).

Constipation

Opioids slow down the gut so constipation can be an ongoing problem for as long as the person is taking these medications.

- Anyone taking opioids should also be taking a bowel stimulant and a laxative to prevent constipation (see Constipation, p.75).
- Tell your home care nurse immediately if there is any change in regular bowel routine.

Confusion

A person who is taking pain medications, especially opioids, may feel a little confused. Some people may even have hallucinations, although this is an unusual response and can be treated.

- If confusion occurs, tell your home care nurse. Lower doses of this medication or use of another type may be recommended. In addition, other aspects of the disease may be causing the confusion and might need to be looked into.

Myoclonus

This is a twitching or spasm of the muscles that the person cannot control.

- Myoclonus is a similar feeling to the one that can occur when you are just about asleep and suddenly jump awake.
- It is not an unusual response to some medications. The twitching is not related at all to a convulsion (see Convulsions, p.100).
- Tell your home care nurse if myoclonus is happening.

Addiction and physical dependence

There is a difference between addiction and physical dependence. Physical dependence is the body's need to maintain the effect of a medication. When the medication is stopped, the body will experience symptoms of withdrawal. Addiction is what some people refer to as psychological dependence - a need to feel a 'high' from the medication or unwillingness to be without the sensation it gives.

- One of the greatest myths about pain management is that people who are taking medications for pain become addicted to them. People do not become addicted to pain medications that are used correctly.
- Research has shown that less than one per cent of hospitalized patients receiving opioids for pain will become addicted. Most people stop taking the opioids when the pain stops.
- Even in the case of chronic pain and long-term opioid use, although physical dependence might occur, addiction is rare.

Tolerance

- Many people taking pain medication will need a higher dose over time because the body develops a tolerance for it.
- The dose of a opioid can be increased as much as necessary by the doctor to relieve pain.

OTHER WAYS TO MANAGE PAIN RELIEF

There are other ways that pain control can sometimes be managed successfully.

TENS (Transcutaneous Nerve Stimulation)

This technique involves using a small electronic device to send weak electric pulses through the skin to the underlying nerves. It is thought that the mild electrical activity helps to stop pain.

- The placing of the electrodes depends on the area and type of pain. A physiotherapist or other member of the health care team who is trained in TENS can teach you where to put the electrodes and how to use the TENS machine.

- The electrodes should not be placed inside an area where radiation is being given at the present, nor for 10 to 14 days afterward.
- TENS should not be used over sinuses, eyes and ears.
- Someone with a pacemaker should not use TENS.
- TENS should not be used near the heart.
- TENS should not be placed on sore, swollen, infected or unhealthy skin.

Other forms of non-medication pain relief

- Some complementary therapies can help distract from pain and may offer pain relief (see Complementary Care, p.87).
- A local anesthetic can be injected around nerves to block pain that is occurring in one area. The results may be temporary or long lasting.
- Acupuncture is an ancient Chinese treatment that uses sterile needles placed at specific places in the body to relieve pain.
- Radiation can be used to shrink tumours to reduce a person's symptoms.
- Neurosurgery, although available, is usually not necessary with the proper use of medication and other techniques.

SKIN PROBLEMS

ITCHING

Itching is an unpleasant sensation that causes a desire to scratch or rub the skin. Common causes of itching during a terminal illness include dry skin, allergy, side effects of medications, chemotherapy or radiation therapy and tumour growth.

What you may expect

A terminal illness can cause many changes in the skin. Some of these changes can be very uncomfortable and may lead to restlessness, anxiety, skin sores and infection.

- Skin may be dry, red, rough, flaky.
- A slight or widespread rash may occur.
- Scratching may cause bleeding and skin sores.

IMPORTANT POINTS

- **Call for help if:**
  - *itching does not disappear after two days.*
  - *the person's skin takes on a yellowish colour.*
  - *the person scratches so much that the skin is raw.*
  - *the rash becomes worse after creams or ointments have been applied.*

How you can offer care

Scratching without thinking or during sleep may be difficult to control. The main comfort you can provide is finding ways to soothe the itching skin.

- Apply skin creams with a water-soluble base two to three times a day, especially after a bath when the skin is damp.
- Use warm water instead of hot for bathing because hot water dries the skin.
- Add baking soda or bath oil to the bath water.
- Wash skin gently using a mild soap. Do not scrub.
- Use baking soda instead of deodorant under the arms.
- Keep nails clean and cut short.
- Encourage the use of rubbing, pressure or vibration instead of scratching.
- Choose loose clothing made of a soft fabric.
- Change bed sheets daily.
- Help keep body fluid levels up by encouraging the person to drink water and other liquids.
- Provide diversions such as television, radio, books.
- Cover the person with lightweight bedding.
- Avoid scented and alcohol-based products on the skin.
- Use gentle detergents for laundry.

BED SORES (PRESSURE SORES)

A bed sore develops when the oxygen flow to a particular area of the body is stopped and the tissue in that area dies. The sores are made worse when the person rubs against the sheets, is pulled up in the bed or chair, or is left with urine or a bowel movement on the skin for too long.

What you need to know

The best approach to bed sores is prevention (see Attention to Pressure Areas, p.33). They are very difficult to heal once they occur. The first hint of a sore is a sign for extra care.

- Red areas on the skin that do not go away, even if the pressure is removed, are a warning that a sore may develop.
- Cracked, blistered, scaly, broken skin can break down very easily.

IMPORTANT POINTS

An open sore on the skin surface or into underlying tissue needs urgent attention.

- **Call for help if:**
  - *you notice cracked, blistered, scaly, broken or reddened skin.*
  - *the sore is getting larger.*
  - *the sore smells foul.*
  - *you notice thick green liquid draining from the sore.*

- Pain at the "pressure points" (back of head, back of shoulders, elbows, buttocks, and heels) are a warning that these areas need special attention. (See figure 26)
- Yellowish-coloured stains on clothing, sheets or chair (could be tinged with blood) are probably from an oozing sore.

How you can offer care

A person who is bedridden, or always in a wheelchair, puts constant pressure on the same places, making these areas more likely to develop sores. If sores develop, they should be kept clean and no further pressure allowed on the area. Tell your home care nurse right away if you find a sore.

- Protect "pressure points" with pillows to help prevent sores. If possible, use sheepskins, heel pads and elbow pads.
- Ask your home care nurse about changing to a mattress that reduces pressure.
- Have the person sit in a chair every day if possible.
- Lift, rather than pull, the person when changing positions.
- Keep sheets pulled tight to prevent wrinkles
- Keep the head of the bed flat or up at a 30-degree angle so there is less pressure at the base of the spine.
- Move the person in bed every two hours from left side, to back, to right side. This turning should be continued every four hours through the night time.
- Change the bed immediately and clean the skin if the person has urine or bowel movement on the skin.
- Encourage the person to eat foods that are high in protein (see Food and Fluid Needs, p. 45).

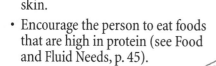

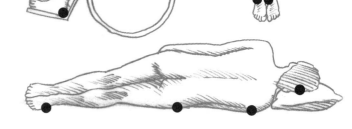

figure 26

MOUTH PROBLEMS

THRUSH (ORAL CANDIDIASIS)

Thrush occurs commonly in people with advanced illness. It is most likely to occur after the person has been on steroids or antibiotics, and is common after radiation of the mouth.

What you need to know

A thrush infection is serious and needs careful attention.

- Your loved one may complain of a sore mouth, sore throat, dry scratchy throat, hoarseness, or problems swallowing.
- When you inspect the mouth, you will see white curd-like patches on the tongue, roof of the mouth, inside cheeks and lips, and back of the throat.
- Thrush is treated with the medication nystatin (such as Mycostatin™, Nadostine™, Nilstat™, Nystex™). The medication is a liquid that is swished in the mouth like a mouth wash, then swallowed.
- The doctor may prescribe a medicated cream to rub on the gums under dentures.
- Thrush can be spread to others. Avoid kissing the person on the lips or sharing utensils if you suspect thrush.

How you can offer care

Before each dose of medication is taken, the mouth should be well cleaned. (See the section Mouth Care, p.30 for guidance on doing this.)

- Tell your home care nurse immediately if you suspect thrush.
- Use a new toothbrush before treatment begins and replace it again when all the medication is finished.
- Help the person rinse well with clear water before taking the medication.
- Remove dentures before medication is taken.
- Clean dentures well at each treatment. If they are not cleaned properly, they can reinfect the mouth.
- Soak the dentures each night in a solution of one part vinegar to four parts water.

MOUTH SORES

Mouth sores are like little cuts or ulcers in the mouth. Chemotherapy, radiation therapy, infection, lack of fluids, poor mouth care, oxygen therapy, too much alcohol or tobacco use, and some medications can cause them.

What you need to know

Mouth sores can be very painful and interfere with eating and drinking.

- Small ulcers or sores in mouth, on gums, or on the tongue may be seen.
- The sores may be red, bleed or have small white patches in the middle.
- The inside of the mouth, gums and tongue may look red, shiny or swollen.
- There may be blood or pus in the mouth.
- A white or yellow film in the mouth may occur.
- Food that is eaten may cause dryness or mild burning.
- There may be sensitivity to hot and cold.
- Increased or decreased mucus in the mouth may be a problem.
- The person may have difficulty swallowing.
- A sore throat or a burning sensation in upper chest may be a symptom.
- To help with pain the doctor may order a product such as Maalox™ or Milk of Magnesia™, with or without xylocaine, that can be painted on sores with a Q-tip™ or swished around the mouth.

How you can offer care

The mouth care you offer helps ease the discomfort with soothing products and non-irritating food and drink.

- Check the mouth twice a day using a small flashlight and tongue blade. If the person wears dentures, remove these first.
- Tell your home care nurse if the person's mouth looks different or there is a change in taste or sensation.
- Do mouth care 30 minutes after eating and every two hours while the person is awake.
- Use one of the suggested rinsing solutions after the mouth care (see Dry Mouth, p.73).
- Apply a water-soluble lubricant such as Muco™ or K-Y Jelly™ to help soothe the lips.
- Encourage the person to drink at least two litres or eight cups of fluid a day.
- Offer small, frequent, cold, non-spicy, bland meals.
- Try chilled foods and fluids (popsicles, ice cubes, frozen yogurt, sherbet, ice cream).

- Avoid citrus fruits and juices such as oranges, lemons, limes, and tomatoes. Although they may seem to moisten the mouth, they actually have a drying effect.

IMPORTANT POINTS

- Always use an ultra-soft toothbrush. A hard brush can damage fragile gum tissue.
- Avoid commercial mouthwashes that contain alcohol. These can all cause more drying and pain.
- Do not use dental floss as it can damage gum tissue.
- Encourage the person to avoid tobacco or alcohol. These can aggravate mouth sores.
- If mouth sores are severe, leave dentures out except for eating.
- Avoid hard and coarse foods such as crackers, raw vegetables, potato chips.
- Call for help if:
  - *the thrush or sores do not improve.*
  - *drinking and swallowing are affected.*
  - *redness and shininess in the mouth lasts for more than 48 hours.*
  - *the temperature goes above normal.*

DRY MOUTH

Dry mouth may occur when a person is not able to drink the usual volume of liquids. This may happen with nausea, vomiting or a lack of appetite. The reduced fluid will cause saliva to dry up. Some medications and mouth breathing can also cause dry mouth.

What you need to know

Dry mouth can be a source of discomfort for a person.

- The complaint may be a dry mouth or a bad taste in the mouth.
- The person's tongue may be red and coated, and lips dry and cracked.

How you can offer care

The most helpful thing you can do is keep your loved one's mouth clean and moist, to help it feel fresh.

- Help the person to clean the mouth often, especially after eating and before bed (see Mouth Care, p.30). One of the rinsing solutions suggested in that section can help moisten the mouth.

- Put a water-soluble lubricant such as Muco™ or K-Y Jelly™ on the lips after cleaning.
- Try a bowl of ice chips by the bed. Even if the person does not want to drink, these can be sucked to moisten the mouth.
- Try a commercial moistening product such as Moistir™ or Oral Balance™.
- Remove dentures, rub a moistening product over the gums, then replace the dentures.
- Do not use commercial mouthwashes that contain alcohol. It causes more drying.

BOWEL AND BLADDER PROBLEMS

INCONTINENCE

Incontinence is lack of control of the bowels or bladder.

What you need to know

For some people, the best choice for controlling incontinence of urine is use of a catheter or condom catheter.

- A catheter is a tube put into the bladder so the urine can drain into a specially designed bag.
- For men, condom catheters fit over the penis and are attached to a collecting bag.

> ## IMPORTANT POINTS
>
> - **Call for help if:**
>   - *there is leaking around where the catheter enters the body.*
>   - *the urine becomes cloudy, has an offensive smell, or the person develops a sudden fever. These could indicate a bladder infection.*
>   - *there is blood in the urine.*
>   - *the person is having diarrhea.*

How you can offer comfort and care

Skin breakdown, which can be caused by pressure and contact with urine or a bowel movement, is a risk from incontinence. For that reason, plus the person's comfort, clean and dry skin is important.

- Consider special incontinence garments (e.g. Stayfree™, DryPlus™, Attends™, Poise™, Ensure Guards™) available at drugstores and supermarkets. They keep the bed dry and should be changed often. Your home care nurse can give you advice about these. You may be able to get financial assistance to cover their cost (see Financial Aid, p.130).

- Use water-repellent creams containing zinc oxide and silicone (e.g. Zincofax™, Penaten Cream™, A&D Cream™) applied as needed to help prevent skin irritation. A silicone and zinc oxide spray (e.g. Silon™) is available and may be easier to use.
- Wash the area where the catheter enters the body at least once a day with soap and water to protect the skin and prevent infection.
- Wash your hands before and after working with the catheter, drainage bag or incontinence garments.
- Check the drainage tubing for kinks and make sure the drainage bag is below the level of the person to encourage draining by gravity.
- Empty the drainage bag at least twice a day.

CONSTIPATION

When a person has a bowel movement, stool (feces) is passed. Constipation means difficulty passing stool. It can be caused by:

- not drinking enough.
- not eating enough.
- not enough fibre in diet.
- decreased physical exercise.
- slowing of the gut due to some medications such as opioids.
- certain illnesses.

What you need to know

Constipation is uncomfortable and may cause serious problems.

- Stool may be dry and painful to pass.

IMPORTANT POINTS

- Keep track of the person's bowel movements. If there has been no bowel movement in two days, contact your home care nurse.
- Avoid bulk laxatives such as Metamucil™. For them to be effective, a person must drink three litres of fluid a day. Otherwise they just make the problem worse.
- Call for help if:
  - there is blood in or around anal area or in stool.
  - there is no bowel movement within one day of taking a laxative.
  - the person has persistent cramps or vomiting.

- The person may have large amounts of gas, burping, or feeling sick to the stomach.
- There may be pain in the abdomen.
- Sometimes there seems to be diarrhea. In fact, it is small amounts of runny stool escaping around the hard stool.
- The person may have small hard bowel movements but not enough stool to correct the constipation.
- Headaches and confusion may accompany constipation.
- The person's abdomen may look blown-up or bloated.

- The doctor may prescribe a stool softener or a laxative. These medications come in the form of a pill or a suppository (see Giving Medications by Suppository, p.57).
- Some people with constipation do not respond to medications or diet changes. They may need an enema.

How you can offer comfort and care

If you are aware of the causes listed above, you may be able to take steps to prevent constipation.

- Try gradually increasing the intake of whole grains in cereals and breads.
- Increase fluid intake to at least two litres or eight to 10 glasses a day.
- Offer a hot drink with caffeine in the morning to encourage a bowel movement.
- Encourage the person to walk, exercise or move about in bed. This might help move stool through the bowel.
- Avoid foods that can cause constipation such as chocolate, cheese and eggs.
- Remind the person of the need to take prescribed stool softeners and laxatives especially if opioids are being used (see Side Effects of Opioids, p.66).
- Offer a variety of fruits (including prunes), vegetables and fruit juices (including prune juice once a day). The following fruit laxative may be a way to encourage the person to take a variety of these helpful foods.

> ### Fruit laxative
> - 1/4 cup currants
> - 1/4 cup raisins
> - 1/4 cup prunes
> - 1/4 cup dates
> - 1/4 cup figs
> - prune juice
>
> *Put first five ingredients in a blender. Add enough prune juice to make a jam-like consistency. Mixture can be eaten by itself, or used as jam, or sauce on ice cream.*

Bowel routine

Anyone using opioids for pain should use a stool softener and a laxative. Also, a basic bowel routine is advised for someone using opioids. Bowel routines must be used daily to work. The following is one suggested routine:

- 1 stool softener such as docusate each morning (e.g. Surfak™, Colace™).
- 1 stool softener each afternoon.
- 2 bowel stimulants (e.g. Senokot™) at bedtime.
  - When taking a stool softener, the person must drink a lot of fluid.
  - Bowel stimulants increase bowel activity and help to create a bowel movement.
  - All can be purchased at the drugstore and their cost may be covered by a drug program (see Financial Aid, p.130).

Enemas

An enema is fluid injected into the rectum to clean out the bowel. To give a small enema such as a Fleet™ the same procedure is followed as for suppositories.

- Help the person into a position that will make it easy to insert the enema tube. The best position is lying on the left side, with the upper leg bent forward. (There will be a diagram on the instructions that come with the enema.)
- Warn the person that the enema may cause a feeling of pressure and cramps.
- The tube will already be lubricated.
- Insert the tube gently into the rectum and squeeze the container.
- Go more slowly but try not to stop if the person has discomfort. The full enema or as much as the person can tolerate should be used.
- Encourage the person to hold the enema in as long as possible before expelling.

DIARRHEA

Diarrhea is the passage of loose or watery bowel movements three or more times a day. There may or may not be discomfort. Causes of diarrhea include infections, some medications, side effects of chemotherapy, radiation therapy to the abdomen, and sometimes the disease itself.

What you need to know

- Diarrhea can upset the balance in the body of salts and chemicals called electrolytes.
- Certain foods can make the diarrhea worse while other foods may help to slow it.
- Dehydration is always a risk in severe diarrhea.
- Diarrhea may be the overflow of liquid stool around hard stool and needs to be treated as constipation (see p.75). Ask your home care nurse about this possibility.

IMPORTANT POINTS

- Foods that may stimulate or irritate the digestive tract should be avoided. Examples are whole grain bread and cereal, fried or greasy food, nuts, raw fruits or vegetables, rich pastries, strong spices and herbs, caffeinated foods or drinks, alcoholic or carbonated beverages, tobacco products.
- Very hot or very cold foods can trigger diarrhea.
- Avoid giving only clear liquids for more than two days in a row.
- **Call for help if:**
  - *the person has six or more loose bowel movements more than two days in a row.*
  - *you notice blood in or around the anal area or in the bowel movement.*

How you can offer comfort and care

If possible, food should be the first choice for restoring the fluid balance of the body.

- Choose foods high in protein, calories and potassium. Talk to your dietitian or home care nurse about suitable foods.
- Encourage the person to drink about two litres or eight to 10 glasses of fluid daily. Sipping slowly will help the fluids to be absorbed better.
- Make sure water is not the only fluid taken. Serve a variety of drinks and jelly products such as Jello™.
- Give frequent small meals instead of three large meals.
- Wash the anal area with mild soap and pat dry after each bowel movement.
- Apply a water-repellent product (Zincofax™, Penaten Cream™, A&D Cream™, Silon™) to the anal area to protect the skin.
- Be calm when the diarrhea occurs. Try to reduce the person's anxiety and embarrassment at the situation.
- Use protective pads on the bed to lessen the person's embarrassment and help with clean-up.
- Use a room deodorizer if odour is a problem.

SHORTNESS OF BREATH
(Dyspnea)

Shortness of breath, also called dyspnea, occurs when the body cannot get enough oxygen. Either the lungs cannot take in enough air, or they cannot deliver enough oxygen to the blood stream. Shortness of breath has many causes including illness, anxiety or pollution (including tobacco smoke).

What you need to know

Severe shortness of breath can be frightening for both the person experiencing it and anyone watching. If you know what to expect, it may be less disturbing.

- The skin around mouth and nailbeds may become blue tinged.
- There may be large amounts of thick mucus that the person can or cannot cough up.
- Respirations may sound moist and gurgling.
- Breathing may be difficult when talking, or even resting.
- Depending on the cause of the shortness of breath, there may be treatment for it.

How you can offer comfort and care

Your loved one may have less trouble breathing if the surroundings are calm and you follow some guidelines.

IMPORTANT POINTS

- **Call for help if:**
  - *the person complains of chest pain.*
  - *thick, yellow, green or bloody mucus is being produced.*
  - *the person cannot get a proper breath for three minutes.*
  - *the skin is pale or blue or the person feels cold and clammy.*
  - *there is a fever.*
  - *the nostrils flare during breathing.*

- Encourage the quiet presence of a family member or friend to help ease the anxiety.
- Plan frequent rest periods between activities if the shortness of breath is worse with movement, washing, dressing or talking.
- Ask visitors just to sit quietly so there is no need to talk.
- Be sure medication prescribed for shortness of breath is taken as directed.
- Use a humidifier to help loosen mucus so coughing is easier.
- Open a window or use a fan to help breathing.
- Remove tight or constricted clothing or bedding and use a lightweight blanket.

- Help the person to a position that makes breathing easier. Lying flat often makes shortness of breath worse. Usually a high sitting position is best. This can be done by putting several pillows at the back. Another helpful position is leaning on a bed table or high table with the head resting on crossed arms.
- Try a recliner chair for sleep as it keeps the body in a semi-upright position.
- Do whatever you can to help the person remain relaxed as tense muscles will add to the breathlessness.

OXYGEN THERAPY

What you need to know

Sometimes the doctor will recommend oxygen therapy to relieve shortness of breath.

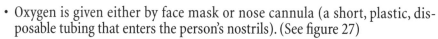

figure 27

- Oxygen is given either by face mask or nose cannula (a short, plastic, disposable tubing that enters the person's nostrils). (See figure 27)
- The mask is plastic and disposable. It fits over the nose and mouth firmly and is attached to the oxygen supply.

How you can offer comfort and care

A mask or cannula needs attention to be as comfortable as possible.

- Remove and clean the mask as needed.
- Place something soft such as small cotton pads or moleskin between the tubing and the skin to lessen irritation.
- Tighten the elastic on a mask enough that it fits snugly on the person's face.
- The prongs of the nasal cannula must be in the person's nose.
- Oxygen can dry the inside of the nose. A water-based, non-prescription preparation can help this. One designed for the problem is Secaris™.

IMPORTANT POINTS

- Oxygen can fuel a fire.
  - *Do not smoke or light matches in a room where oxygen is in use.*
  - *Do not use oxygen around a gas stove.*
  - *Do not use oil-based products such as Vaseline™ or mineral oil close to oxygen.*
- Use oxygen only as the doctor directs. This may be 24 hours a day or only sometimes.
- Oxygen is needed most during activity such as getting in and out of the tub, on outings, when walking.
- Make sure a 24 hour supply of oxygen is available, especially on weekends.
- Follow the supplier's instructions to ensure that the equipment works properly.
- Know the number of the supplier to call if you have a problem.

NAUSEA AND VOMITING

Nausea means feeling sick to the stomach and vomiting means throwing up. Nausea can happen even when a person is not thinking about food. Vomiting can occur even if nothing has been eaten or there has been no nausea.

Many things can cause nausea and vomiting. These include illness, medications, irritation of the digestive system, certain foods, constipation and movement. Sometimes the cause has nothing to do with the terminal illness and is as simple as the flu.

What you need to know

Everyone has experienced nausea and vomiting at some time. The difference for a person with a terminal illness may be its frequency and intensity, made worse by the weakness that accompanies the illness.

- The person may feel sick and unable to eat.
- Vomiting may be occasional or often.
- Medications taken by mouth may be vomited.
- The person may be comfortable at rest but feel sick with movement.

IMPORTANT POINTS

- Position a person who is in bed and vomiting on the side so the vomit will not be inhaled and the person will not choke.
- Keep a record of how often and how much the person vomits.
- Medications used to treat motion sickness (such as Gravol™) make a person sleepy and are not recommended.
- **Call for help if:**
  - *the vomiting occurs more than three times an hour for three or more hours.*
  - *blood or material that looks like coffee grounds appears in the vomit.*
  - *the person is not able to take in more than four cups of liquid or ice chips in a day or is not able to eat solid foods for two days.*
  - *medications are vomited.*
  - *the person feels unusually weak and dizzy.*
  - *the person loses consciousness.*

How you can offer comfort and care

The comfort you can offer is aimed mostly at reducing any of the triggers that might cause the nausea and vomiting, and providing medications to control it.

- Focus on providing favourite foods in small quantities.
- Try offering small amounts of food often.
- Encourage the person to take the anti-nausea medication regularly.
- Ask your home care nurse about other ways medications can be given such as by suppository or with a patch on the skin.
- Freshen the mouth with a non-alcohol based mouthwash or club soda.
- Remove the basin with vomit in it right away. Keep a clean basin close by.
- Open windows or use a fan to see if fresh air will help reduce the nausea.
- Try cold foods because they have less odour.
- Keep a supply of clear fluids, ice chips, frozen juice chips, and ginger ale to offer in small quantities.
- Cooking smells can increase nausea so try to keep these away from the sick person.
- Do not offer greasy or spicy foods. Try bland foods such as crackers, toast, angel food cake, soft fruits and yogurt.
- Help the person to rest sitting up for an hour after meals.
- Encourage anyone who will be close to the person to avoid using perfumes, after-shaves or deodorants with strong fragrances.
- Ask your doctor, home care nurse or pharmacist if some of the complementary care suggestions such as herbal remedies would help (see Herbal Remedies, p.94).

TROUBLE SLEEPING
(Insomnia)

Insomnia means the inability to sleep properly when sleep would normally be expected. It may range from a disturbed sleep to being fully awake.

What you may expect

At some time or another, most people who are dying have difficulty falling asleep or staying asleep.

- Insomnia can be caused by anxiety, fear, sadness or other psychological or spiritual concerns.
- Physical problems such as pain, nausea, vomiting and coughing may cause insomnia.

IMPORTANT POINTS

- Do not ignore the person's pain, nausea or coughing. Give medications that have been prescribed.
- Call for help if:
  - the person becomes confused at nighttime.
  - you are not sleeping and need relief.

How you can offer comfort and care

A person who has a terminal illness may sleep a lot during the day. Then, at the usual times for sleep, insomnia seems to be a problem.

- Allow the person to sleep whenever, and as much as needed, without staying to a schedule.
- Provide warm, non-caffeine drinks such as warm milk with honey before sleep.
- Spend quiet times with the person, listening and talking. The opportunity to express feelings will do much to relieve a person's emotional concerns.
- Try to make the person comfortable. Sometimes if you lie on the bed beside the person, your close contact will give comfort.
- Give backrubs or massage the person's feet for relaxation.
- Keep sheets clean, neatly tucked in and as free from wrinkles as possible.
- Be sure the area is quiet when the person wants to sleep.

SWELLING (Edema)

Edema is extra fluid in the tissues or in the abdomen. It may occur if the body retains salt or water, or is poorly nourished. Also too little protein in the body, tumours and obstruction to the veins or lymph system may cause edema. Unless the swelling is related to a heart problem, water pills will not be effective to remove the extra fluid.

What you may expect

When fluid accumulates in the abdomen or elsewhere, some easily identified changes take place.

- The feet and lower legs swell when the person sits, stands or walks.
- Rings become too tight for the fingers.
- The person complains of "tightness" in hands when making a fist.
- The abdomen looks distended or blown up, or the person may complain of tight pants.

How you can offer comfort and care

Everything you can do to reduce edema is directed toward preventing fluid accumulating in the outer limbs.

- Encourage bed rest with feet up on two pillows.
- When in a chair, keep the person's feet elevated on a stool with a pillow. If the arms are swollen, they can be kept elevated by resting them on a table, cushioned on a pillow.
- Massage the swollen areas to help the fluid be absorbed.

IMPORTANT POINTS

- **Call for help if:**
  - *you press your finger into the swollen area and the finger mark stays.*
  - *the swelling spreads up legs or arms.*
  - *the swelling in the belly causes the person to become short of breath.*

LOSS OF STRENGTH

Loss of strength may be a result of the advancing illness or may be from weakened muscles after a prolonged stay in bed. It usually occurs gradually but sometimes can happen over just a few days.

What you may expect

A person who used to be active and independent will usually have difficult times adjusting to the physical limitations of an illness. If you understand how weakness affects the body, you can plan your care accordingly.

- Tiredness is common after activities that once were easy.
- The person may need help to walk, bath or dress, or may need to be cared for in bed.
- It may be difficult for the person to move in bed and get from one place to another.
- Frustration with physical limitations may make the person irritable over situations that would normally pass unnoticed.

How you can offer comfort and care

Your care will focus on helping your loved one save energy during activities.

- Ask a member of the health care team to teach you techniques for helping a person move more easily.
- Reassure the person that you are happy to help. Someone who is losing strength often becomes upset about being dependent.
- Put a bell, a spoon and tin plate, or anything that can be used to make a noise so you can be called when needed. Baby monitors work well.
- Remind the person about the need to limit activities and to rest before doing anything strenuous.
- Ask a member of your health care team about obtaining a walker or wheelchair to make movement around the home safer and easier. You can buy or rent these and they are also available from Alberta Aids to Daily Living (AADL).

CONFUSION

A person who has trouble thinking and acting appropriately or has disturbed thought is said to be confused. A seriously ill person may become confused due to the illness, infection, a side effect of medications, or lack of fluids. Tell your home care nurse if you notice the person starting to be confused. There is often something that can be done to help.

What you need to know

Confusion often goes hand-in-hand with a physical illness. If you understand how a confused person may act, you will be less anxious when you see unfamiliar behaviours.

- Confusion can start very slowly.
- There may be poor concentration, loss of memory and of interest.
- Decision-making may be difficult because of poor concentration.
- Sometimes there is a sense of unreality or of going crazy.
- Feelings may fluctuate between denial and acceptance of the situation.
- A confused person may become restless and move about in a random fashion. There may appear to be pain.
- The person may see or hear things that are not real (hallucinations), particularly at night.
- Strange thoughts may bother the person.
- Fear and anger may be present for no obvious reason.
- Movements may become slowed.
- If the confusion becomes so severe that the person cannot make proper decisions, you may need to take legal responsibility for affairs (see Legal Affairs, Appendix II, p.133).

How you can offer comfort and care

Since harm can come easily to a confused person, supervision and guidance are needed.

- Remind the person who you are whenever this seems necessary.
- Touch the person during conversations as a reminder you are there. Stand face to face and stay within a few feet of the person when talking.
- Turn off radio and TV when you are talking. Do not play them together or loudly.
- Talk slowly and use short statements.

- Keep a calendar and clock in view and remind often what day and time it is.
- Keep the room well-lit.
- Do not give medications or any care without explaining what you are doing.
- Do not leave the person alone for long periods.
- Use bedrails to reduce the chance of the person falling out of bed.

IMPORTANT POINTS

● **Call for help if:**
- *confusion occurs very suddenly or becomes worse.*
- *the person becomes violent or very agitated.*
- *you or the person is hurt because of the confusion.*
- *you are tired and need relief.*

COMPLEMENTARY CARE

The word complementary suggests care techniques that are used along with conventional medicine. The ones described here are some that you might use in your home to help your loved one feel more comfortable. They are not intended as a substitute for medical care and you should never use them without checking first with a member of your health care team. There are other types of complementary care available that you may want to explore and your home care nurse can discuss these with you.

RELAXATION TECHNIQUES

Since the main purpose of relaxation aids is to focus your loved one on the activity and away from the discomfort of the illness, anything you can do to provide distraction is helpful. **Never** use relaxation techniques as a substitute for pain relief medications.

How you can offer comfort

Techniques for relaxation involve a conscious attempt to relax all the muscles. These are more structured than we usually mean when we think of relaxing. All relaxation techniques begin in the same way.

- Choose a quiet room.
- Try to avoid interruptions during the time of the chosen activity. Hang a "Do Not Disturb" sign on the door if need be.

- Choose a time that feels right. Some times could be:
  - before the pain or discomfort is severe.
  - when the person feels worried or nervous.
  - at the same time every day.
- Ask if there is any music that would offer added relaxation.
- Help the person settle into a comfortable position, with arms and legs relaxed.
- Have the person begin the activity by breathing in deeply through the nose and out slowly through the mouth, as though whistling. This should be done three times. Do not encourage a person with breathing problems to do deep breathing exercises.
- Encourage the person to keep eyes closed and focus on how the activity feels.
- Have the person think of a calm, peaceful place and picture the body being very light, floating, or nice and warm.
- Ask for feedback after the activity so you know what is successful and what is not.

Imagery

Imagery relaxation is use of the imagination to help someone relax. It is a way of "picturing" something to take the mind off discomfort.

What you do

- Remind the person of the preparation for relaxation techniques.
- Provide ideas for images of pain relief. For example:
  - view pain as a large rock that is part of the body, then a large helium balloon is tied to the rock, taking the rock and the pain away.
  - feel pain as a thunderstorm that rains on the body, then a gentle breeze blows the thunderstorm and the pain away.
  - remember a special place where the person has been that creates its own images.
  - Help the person do the imagery relaxation 20 minutes a day.

Relaxation breathing

Relaxation breathing is a technique of breathing in a controlled way to relax tense muscles and take the mind off discomfort.

What you need

- Cassette player (with or without headphones)
- Relaxation tapes to help the person work through the relaxation breathing.

What you do

- Remind the person of the preparation for relaxation techniques.
- Make the relaxation tape the focus of the exercise.
- The breathing exercises are done in a rotation.
  - Breathe in deeply through the nose, at the same time tensing a muscle or group of muscles. For example make a fist or clench teeth.
  - Hold the breath and tense muscles for one to two seconds.
  - Relax the muscles and breathe out slowly.
  - Tense the muscles in the lower right leg while breathing in deeply.
  - Relax the muscles in the lower right leg while breathing out slowly.
  - Repeat with the lower left leg, then slowly work the way up the body. Each time, tense the muscles while breathing in deeply and relax while breathing out slowly.
- Encourage these exercises at least 20 minutes a day.
- Avoid relaxation tapes that may cause bad or worrying thoughts.
- Have a person who has problems breathing just relax for a minute or two before the exercises instead of doing the deep breathing.

VIBRATION MASSAGE

Vibration massage is a massage using an electric device. It helps to numb the area of pain and to relax tense muscles.

What you need

- Electric massager

What you do

- Choose the area of the body where there is pain.
- Remove clothing from the area.
- Cover areas not being massaged, for warmth and privacy.
- Find positions in which you will both be comfortable.
- Massage an area below or above the pain if the actual area is too painful to touch.
- Try using the massager on the other side of the body from an area of pain. For instance if the right hip hurts, try the massager on the left hip.
- Do not do vigorous massage over the area of a tumour.
- Apply the massager for 25 to 45 minutes, twice a day.
- Turn the massager on and off every few seconds for 25 to 45 minutes if that is more comfortable.
- Follow the instructions on the electric massager to avoid electrical shock.

DISTRACTION

Any technique that helps distract a person from the immediate discomfort can be helpful. Begin by preparing the area as you would for relaxation techniques.

Music

Music has the power to absorb some people so totally that they forget everything else for a while. With headphones to block out other sounds, the distraction can be even more complete.

What you need
- Radio, CD or cassette player (with or without headphones)
- CDs or cassettes of the music the person likes

What you do
- Help the person choose some favourite music.
- Encourage singing along with the music, or keeping time by tapping with fingers and feet to the beat.
- Try using music distraction several times a day.

Humour

Laughter can lift a person's mood and even ease pain. Humour distraction helps your loved one focus on something other than the discomfort.

What you need
- Cassette player
- Comedy audio or video tapes
- VCR
- Television
- Radio

What you do
- Find out what type of humour the person is in a mood for - maybe British comedy or slapstick.
- Help with the choice of a comedy audio or video tape.

COMFORT FROM COLD TREATMENTS

Cold applied to the body has many benefits. It reduces muscles spasms, numbs nerve endings, reduces swelling and eases itching.

- Cold that is to be left in one place, rather than massaged over an area, should be wrapped in a cloth.
- Leave the cold on for at least 10 to 15 minutes. It can be left on for up to 30 minutes.
- Do this three to four times a day.
- Switch back and forth from cold to heat if that provides comfort.
- Try applying heat rubs and ointments such as Ben Gay™, Rub A.535™, Tiger Balm™ to the painful area before using the ice cold treatment.
  - Do not use a cold rub cream such as Icy Cold™ at the same time as any other cold treatment.
  - Test creams or ointments on the inside of an arm first to be sure they do not irritate the skin. If there is no redness or itching after a few minutes, try it on the area of pain.
  - Wash your hands after putting on creams. Be sure you do not get any cream near your eyes.

Ice bags

These are bags used to apply cold to a painful area.

What you need

- Ice bag made up from one of the following:
  - commercial ice bag
  - Ziploc™ bag filled with crushed or shaved ice
  - bag containing small pieces of frozen food such as corn, peas or unpopped popcorn kernels.
- Towel or pillowcase
- Heat rub (optional)

What you do

- Push all the air from the bag if using a Ziploc™ bag filled with ice.
- Hit a bag of frozen vegetables on the counter top to break them up.
- Place the ice bag in a pillowcase or towel. If the person wants it colder, wet the covering.
- Place the ice bag on the area with pain. If this causes more pain, put the ice bag above or below the area.
- Refreeze the bag of vegetables after use, making sure to mark the bag so you do not use them for eating.

Cold cloths

Cold cloths are simply applied to a painful area.

What you need
- Two towels
- Ice
- Basin
- Heat rub (optional)

What you do
- Fill the basin with 2 inches of water.
- Add ice to the water.
- Soak the towels in the ice water.
- Wring out a towel and put it on the area that hurts.
- When the towel becomes warm, put it back in the ice water and repeat with the second towel.

Cold or ice massage

This is massaging ice or cold onto a painful area.

What you need
- Ice
- Towel and wash cloth
- Plastic bag or garbage bag
- Paper cup

What you do
- Fill a paper cup halfway with water.
- Put the cup in the freezer until the water is frozen solid.
- Peel the cup to uncover the ice.
- Cover the plastic bag with the towel and put under the area that will be massaged to catch the water as it melts.
- Wrap a wash cloth around the paper cup to stop your hands from getting cold.
- Rub the ice in a circle over the area that hurts.
- Dry the skin with the towel as the ice melts.
- Massage the area for about four minutes. It is normal for the area to get red.

COMFORT FROM HEAT TREATMENTS

Heat can be soothing and also has beneficial effects by relaxing tense muscles. There are two important things to remember.

- Use caution when using electric heating pads. They do not turn off and can cause burns.
- Do not use heat rubs when using heat treatments.

Hot water bottles

Most households have a hot water bottle and it can be used with little preparation.

What you do

- Fill the bottle with water from the hot water tap. Do not use boiling water as it may be difficult to judge how hot the bottle will become.
- After putting in the stopper, shake the bottle gently to be sure it will not leak.
- Cover the bottle with a towel or similar cover so there is no direct contact with skin.
- Prop it against the area where the person is having discomfort.

Microwave heat bags

These are bags that can be heated in the microwave and are used to put heat on an area.

What you need

- Microwave
- Flax seed bag or specially formulated heat pack
- Fleece cover or a towel

How you do it

- Put the bag in the microwave and microwave on high for 2 minutes.
- Wrap the bag in the fleece cover or towel. Never use a hot pack without a cover.
- Put the bag on the area that hurts.
- If this causes pain, you can put the bag:
- above or below the area that hurts.
- on the opposite side of the body. For instance if the right leg is sore, try the bag on the left leg.
- Cover the area with blankets to keep the heat in.

IMPORTANT POINTS

There are some points to be aware of when using cold or hot treatments.

- Do not use massage, cold or heat on skin that:
  - *is being radiated.*
  - *is open or has sores.*
  - *you have been told has poor blood flow.*
  - *has bleeding or bruising.*
- Do not use massage, cold or heat if they increase the pain.
- Do not use cold or heat on any area where the person has no sensation (feeling).

HERBAL REMEDIES

You and your loved one may be considering a herbal remedy to help with an effect of the terminal illness. There are some important things you must remember.

- Herbs have been used for centuries to treat and prevent disease. Some of them do have healthful properties, but they may not be appropriate at the time.
- Many people believe that because herbs are "natural," they cannot cause harm. This is simply not true. Herbs are medications in plant form, and have the same potential to cause side effects that other medicines do.
- Herbs can interact with some prescription medications. It is important that you tell your home care nurse, doctor or pharmacist if the person you are caring for is using herbal products and ask about any product if you are uncertain.
- Make sure that any herbs being used are quality products. Most quality products have been tested to ensure they contain a certain percentage of the key ingredient. Also, quality products may have a drug identification number (DIN) and the product must have an expiry date and a lot number.
- Avoid any product about which you have doubts.

Complications that might happen

For some readers, the complications described in this section may be disturbing. They will not necessarily occur in all cases. If one or more of these complications is something that your loved one may experience, your doctor or home care nurse will advise you. The information is included to assist you in being prepared to provide the necessary care if, or when, needed.

COMPLICATIONS FROM PAIN MEDICATIONS
(Opioid Toxicity)

All the food, water or medications that you take into your body are either useable or waste. Your liver does the job of breaking the parts down and your lungs, bowels and kidneys get rid of the waste. Someone who is on high doses or long term opioid pain relief, or has kidney problems may have wastes from the medication build up in the body. This is called opioid toxicity.

What you should know

With opioid toxicity, the person has very marked behaviour changes. There are some signs that you should be aware of if your loved one is using opioids for pain relief.

- Delirium or confusion may be seen in the form of:
  - agitation
  - bad dreams, nightmares
  - decreased level of consciousness, drowsiness
  - confusion about time and place
  - hallucinations (seeing, feeling or hearing things that are not real)
  - moaning and rambling speech
  - reduced concentration
  - restlessness
  - short term memory difficulty
  - sleeping during the day and waking during the night
  - jerking or seizure-like movements of limbs or face muscles
  - seizures
  - pain when touched in a way not expected to cause pain
- If you notice any of these changes, tell your home care nurse.
- A member of your health care team may ask questions to check the person's memory and recognition, so that early signs of the complication can be identified.

How you can offer care

Prevention

- The person must not become dehydrated so the kidneys can keep flushing the wastes out of the body. Either the person must drink many fluids or hypodermoclysis may be considered (see Hypodermoclysis, p.52).
- The doctor may switch opioids. Different opioids make different wastes. By switching from one to another the body can continue to get rid of the wastes.
- If the kidneys are not working properly, the doctor may lower the dose of opioid.

Treatment

- The doctor may order a medication to control hallucinations, nightmares or agitation until the body gets rid of the wastes.

> ## IMPORTANT POINTS
> - **Call for help:**
>   - *if you see any of the signs of opioid toxicity.*

SPINAL CORD COMPRESSION

Spinal cord compression means the spinal cord is being squeezed. It is usually caused by a tumour pressing on the spinal cord. If left untreated, it can paralyze.

What you need to know

About five per cent of people with cancer will develop a cord compression. The most common types of cancer to cause this problem are lung, breast, prostate, multiple myeloma and renal cell.

- The first sign of cord compression is back pain.
- As the compression becomes more severe, the signs include:
  - changes in sensation such as tingling, numbness, pins and needles, hot and cold.
  - bowel and bladder changes - either incontinence or problems passing urine or stool.
  - motor changes - problems getting up, feelings of weakness and no strength in limbs.
  - frequent falls.
- If caught early, radiation therapy and steroid medications can relieve the pressure on the spinal cord and maybe prevent paralysis.

IMPORTANT POINTS

- Tell your home care nurse and doctor immediately if the person starts having signs of a cord compression.

SUPERIOR VENA CAVA SYNDROME

A syndrome is a collection of symptoms all associated with one problem. The symptoms of superior vena cava syndrome are caused by a tumour pressing on the major blood vessel that goes to the heart.

What you need to know

Early signs

In the early stages, some of the following signs may be seen:

- shortness of breath
- fast breathing
- fast heart beat
- headache, dizziness
- standing out of neck and chest veins
- redness of face, neck and upper trunk

> **IMPORTANT POINTS**
> - **Call for help:**
>   - *from your doctor or home care nurse if the person has signs of superior vena cava syndrome.*

Later signs

As the condition progresses, you may notice:

- swelling of the face
- swelling around the eyes
- tightness of collars and jewellery such as rings
- chest pain
- tightness of the throat, difficulty swallowing
- cough
- problem with vision
- arm swelling

CONVULSIONS (Seizures)

Convulsions are seizures or fits that cause loss of consciousness and a jerking movement of muscles. They are caused by changes in the normal nerve impulses to and from the brain. High fever, certain medications, injury to the head, infection of spinal fluid or fluid surrounding the brain, or a tumour in the spine or brain all could result in seizures.

What you need to know

Convulsions can be frightening, especially if you have not seen them before. They will stop on their own after a few seconds or minutes.

- The person cries or moans, then loses consciousness.
- The eyes stare blankly or roll back.
- There may be sudden loss of control of bladder and bowels.
- Jerking movements of the body, especially the arms and legs, occurs.
- The seizure may involve the whole body or just one part.
- If there is a possibility of a convulsion, the doctor may order a medication to help prevent it.

IMPORTANT POINTS

- Do not leave the person during a seizure, not even to call the doctor.
- Never forcefully turn the neck or a rigid limb.
- Never restrain the person's movements.
- Do not move the person except out of danger from a radiator, glass door, stairway or other hazard.
- Do not try to open the person's mouth during the seizure, even if the tongue is being bitten. Keep your hands and fingers away from the person's mouth.
- Wait until the person is fully conscious before giving food, drink or medication.
- Once the seizure is over and the person is comfortable, call the doctor.
- **Call for help if:**
  - *a seizure lasts more than five minutes.*
  - *the person does not regain consciousness when the seizure stops.*
  - *this is the first time a seizure has occurred.*

How you can offer care

Remain calm. Once a seizure has started you cannot make it stop.

- Prevent a fall to the floor by cradling the person in your arms if the seizure occurs while the person is in bed or a chair.
- Move objects that might injure the person.
- Remove eyeglasses and loosen tight clothing.
- Do not try to restrain movement. Let the seizure happen.
- Try to turn the head to the side so saliva can flow out of the mouth, not down the throat.
- Do not try to force open the jaw or put a hard object into the mouth to keep it open. This is dangerous. You may damage the teeth or gums. Also the person may break whatever you use in the mouth and may choke.
- Try to notice what type of movement the person makes, how long the seizure lasts and which parts of the body move with the seizure.
- Stay with the person until the seizure stops. When it does, make sure the breathing is all right.
- Speak gently and reassuringly as the person may be confused or frightened and likely will not remember what happened.
- Be aware that convulsions are exhausting. The person may have a headache and will be very tired and need rest.
- Use side rails and bumper pads on the bed if someone may have seizures. Stay close when the person is walking or sitting in a chair.

HEMORRHAGE

Hemorrhaging is excessive bleeding that is very difficult to stop. It is rare but can happen with certain medical conditions. Stomach or bowel tumours, or tumours that are weakening arteries may cause this bleeding.

What you should know

A hemorrhage can be very frightening both for you and the person who is bleeding. There are some signs that might warn you about the possibility of hemorrhage.

- The person may begin to complain of feeling tired or weak and may be in pain.
- The breathing may become rapid and irregular and the heart rate may increase.
- The person's skin will feel cold and clammy and be pale. These are signs of shock which is the body's reaction to severe hemorrhage.
- If your doctor or nurse thinks the person may hemorrhage, the doctor can order a medication that will make the person drowsy and unaware of what is happening.
- The person may start to bleed out of a tumour, the mouth, nose, ears, rectum or vagina. Sometimes blood does not escape the body but pools inside. When this happens, large bruises will eventually appear on the skin.

How you can offer comfort and care

Hemorrhaging can happen very suddenly, leaving you with little time to respond.

- Discuss with your doctor or home care nurse how you should manage this emergency if it occurs.
- Stay with the person to offer reassurance. Talk calmly and use extra blankets for warmth.
- Do not force someone to stay awake. This will only add to stress and anxiety.
- If blood begins to escape from the body, do not try to stop it. Collect it with dark towels. These will absorb the blood and hide the amount of blood being lost - a cause of anxiety for both you and the person.

As life ends

DYING AT HOME

There are some things you must consider if your loved one plans to die at home.

What you need to consider

The decision to die at home may be a difficult one for both of you to make. Helping someone die at home can be rewarding and is hard work. You need to agree that this is what you both desire.

- Talk to the dying person about the arrangements, and your concerns and feelings.
- Plan for what you will do if you or your loved one has a change of mind about a home death. This is not a failure. You can still help give basic care in a nursing home or hospice and be sure that the person is comfortable.
- Discuss your decision with your home care nurse and doctor.
- Learn what you might expect during the last days of your loved one's life so that you are prepared for the changes you might see.
- Tell your home care nurse about religious or other cultural facts that will be important to you and the dying person.

How you can offer comfort and care

Your role is offering comfort in any way you can.

- Give medicine for pain, nausea and shortness of breath on a regular schedule.
- Play music or read to your loved one if these seem to be relaxing. (Bear in mind that if the person is not fully conscious, it might not be a good idea to play continuous music as the person has no way to shut out the sound.)
- Turn the person every two hours, or rearrange the position with pillows.
- Give back rubs, and maintain skin moisture with lotion.
- Moisten the person's lips, and use lip cream to prevent dryness.
- Be aware of external sounds such as children laughing and determine if these are comforting or upsetting.
- Control the number of visitors and their length of stay so the person does not become exhausted.
- Encourage visitors to phone in advance and tell them if it is not a good time to come.
- If you have a spiritual leader, keep that person aware of your loved one's progress.

Practical details
- Keep the phone numbers of home care nurses and doctors nearby.
- Keep information about care and people to call in a single notebook.
- Prepare a list of people to call near or at the time of death.
- Decide if a spiritual leader should be called before or at the time of death.
- Ask about the doctor attending at the time of death. Since the doctor is not required to come following an expected home death, prior arrangements can be made.

IMPORTANT POINTS

- Instructions not to perform any heroic measures need to be communicated clearly. This means if an ambulance is needed to transport the person to a hospital or a hospice, resuscitation will not be done if the person dies in the ambulance. These instructions may be called a Do Not Resuscitate order (DNR), code status or levels of care. Discuss this with your home care nurse or doctor to make the necessary arrangements.
- Tell people who sit with the person or provide nursing care that calling 911 is not what you and the dying person want.
- Make funeral arrangements with a funeral home and tell them that you are planning a home death.
- If you feel that you cannot go on caring for the person at home, talk to your home care nurse.
- **Call for help if the person:**
  - *is uncomfortable.*
  - *is having trouble breathing.*
  - *seems upset or restless, even if asleep or in a coma.*
  - *has problems passing urine or with bowel movements.*
  - *has fallen.*
  - *is not taking medications.*

A MOVE TO HOSPICE OR HOSPITAL

There may come a time when your loved one needs to be admitted to a care facility or hospital because of physical symptoms related to the illness or because care can no longer be managed.

What you need to remember

Being a caregiver is physically and emotionally challenging. Do not feel a failure if you decide you can no longer provide care at home.

- Continue to stay involved with the person's care either by helping make decisions or by helping with simple tasks.
- Give yourself permission to take time away from the person and go back to your home.
- Ask family or friends to stay with the person if you are uncomfortable leaving.
- Ask for comfortable sleeping arrangements if you wish to spend the night.
- Take a book or some activity to do while you sit with the person.

How you can offer support

The decision to move away from familiar surroundings is never easy for anyone. For someone with a terminal illness, the decision may seem very final.

- Discuss with the person, the decision to move, explaining the limitations you may feel about your ability to give care.
- Involve the person in decisions about anticipated care in the hospital or hospice.
- Be with the person during the move.
- Take meaningful objects from home such as family pictures, a quilt, a pillow and clothes to help make the surroundings familiar.

LAST DAYS OF LIFE

In the final days before death, a person goes through changes as the body gradually shuts down. The person may become withdrawn and less aware of surroundings.

What you may expect

Withdrawal

Someone who is dying feels a separation from the world and may feel that no one really understands the experience. Many religious people experience the anguish of an apparent absence of a spiritual power.

- Many things such as life history, regrets, relationship barriers, losses and thoughts of the after-life become important.
- The person may start to recall memories of people who have died.
- Although the person may appear to have given up, behind the silence there may be many thoughts going on that help deal with the impending death.
- With withdrawal comes less of a need to communicate with others.
- Touch and silence take on more meaning as words lose their importance. This does not mean that the person does not benefit from hearing your words.

Changing levels of awareness

Advanced illness can affect a person's ability to think clearly and respond to surroundings. Mental changes often coincide with the physical changes in the final days of an illness.

- The person may become restless, excited or irritable for no apparent reason.
- Simple directions may be misunderstood.
- Clear thinking and the ability to communicate thoughts may be diminished.
- Familiar people or objects may not be recognized or simple things forgotten.
- Hallucinations may be troublesome.
- The person may be drowsy all the time and fall asleep even during conversations.
- Sometimes the person may appear to be reaching out and even call the name of someone who has died.

How you can offer comfort and care

During the last days of life, the following suggestions may help soothe a person who is withdrawn or disturbed.

- Sit quietly as a comforting presence. Use gentle touch as a reminder that you are there or if you want to speak.
- Move close and talk gently. Assume you can be heard even if you do not get a response.
- Reduce confusion by limiting noisy distractions such as television and radio.
- Ask visitors to talk quietly.
- Gently remind the person of the time, who you are and where you both are.
- Do not argue if reality is different for a dying person. Sometimes agreeing with someone who is mildly confused allows the situation to pass without creating upset.
- Listen quietly if the person needs to express thoughts, worries or feelings.
- Try using soft music for a relaxing effect.
- Continue to offer drinks and very small portions of favourite foods that are soft and easy to eat.
- Take the food away without a fuss if the person refuses anything. Try again later.

SIGNS THAT DEATH IS APPROACHING

What you need to know

As death is near, the body undergoes changes. If you know what to expect, you will be less anxious when you see them happening.

- Respirations change, becoming shallow, quicker or slower.
- Breathing may be difficult, with intermittent periods of no breath.
- Bubbling or rattling sounds in the throat and chest may accompany breathing.
- Swallowing may become difficult.
- Heartbeat may be irregular.
- Anxiety and restlessness may increase.
- There may be a reduced level of consciousness.
- The person has no interest in taking drinks.
- There is a small quantity of very dark urine or no urine at all.
- There is progressive coldness and purple discoloration, mostly in arms and legs.

How you can offer comfort and care

Even if your loved one does not seem to be aware of you during this last stage, your presence is still a comfort.

- Continue to touch and reassure the person that you are close by and you care.
- Speak calmly and naturally.
- Provide comfort by keeping the person dry and lips moistened with a lubricant.
- Raise the head of the bed if breathing is difficult or raise the upper body with pillows.

WHEN DEATH OCCURS

What you need to know

At the time of death, body functions stop.

- There will be no response, no breathing and no pulse.
- The eyes will be fixed in one direction; they may be open or closed.
- The jaws will relax and mouth may be open slightly.
- There may be loss of control of bladder or bowels.

IMPORTANT POINTS

- Even though your loved one may appear to be in distress with difficult breathing and an irregular heartbeat, these may not be troublesome and the person may be very comfortable.
- Do not try to force liquids or food. This can cause choking.
- Continue to give pain medications. Anything you can do to ease the pain and discomfort is important in these last few hours.
- If the person cannot swallow pills, ask the home care nurse for advice.
- Some of the complementary therapies suggested on page 87 may be comforting at this time.
- Even if your loved one appears to be sleeping or unconscious, your words may be understood. Do not say anything you would not want them to hear.

What you do

When death occurs, you may feel an urgency to "do something" but there is no rush.

- **Do not call 911 or an emergency team.** A crew would arrive expecting to save a life or give aggressive treatment. Ambulance crews are bound by law to do this unless a Do Not Resuscitate order is in place.
- Do not feel that you must call the funeral home immediately after the death. Sometimes, friends and family who were not present at death want to see the person.
- Be supportive of anyone who chooses to hug, caress or bathe the person. These are all normal ways of working through the finality of death.
- Call your home care nurse and family doctor to let them know that death has occurred.

How you care for the body

Physical changes take place in the hours after death. Some things can be done to counteract these changes.

- Make sure your loved one is lying on the back with the head slightly elevated by a pillow.
- Close the eyes.
- Put dentures that have been removed back in the mouth immediately.
- Place a small facecloth or towel rolled up under the chin to help keep the jaw closed.
- Remove rings and jewelry unless you all have agreed otherwise. Tape rings if they are to be left on, as the muscles relax later and the rings may slip off.
- Cover the body with a sheet to keep it warm and help decrease stiffness that may occur.
- Have wigs or other appliances ready to go with the person to the funeral home.

How you can comfort yourself and loved ones

There is no hurry.

- If you have a spiritual leader, ask that person to be with you and conduct appropriate farewell rituals at the bedside.
- Family and friends may find it helpful to gather around your loved one and take a moment to express your thanks (aloud or silently) for the person's life. A farewell gesture of a hug, a kiss or a significant spiritual gesture can help to honour the moment and bring closure.
- Be in physical contact with others if that gives you comfort.
- Do things that calm you such a having a warm drink or breathing deeply.
- Spend as much time with your loved one as you wish. Take time to say your good-byes.
- Remember that it may be distressing for you or other family members to be present when your loved one is taken to the funeral home. You may find it easier to be out of the house at that time.

ARRANGEMENTS AFTER DEATH

Arrangements after a death are emotional tasks that are often done when you are least able to think about such decisions. Some people choose to make arrangements in advance. Then, at death there is time to visit with family and begin mourning without worrying about organizational details. For other people, making arrangements in advance seems too final an action and it is more important to enjoy the time with a loved one. There is no correct or incorrect way to do the planning.

ADVANCE PLANNING OF ARRANGEMENTS

What you need to consider
- If you choose to join a memorial society, that organization can help you with advance planning and make all arrangements when death occurs.
- Planning in advance gives you more time to make decisions about the details involved.
- You may save money if you visit several funeral homes and find one that meets your particular needs.
- Pre-paying for a funeral may help defray the costs.
- There is time for everyone to plan a service together before the death occurs. Some people choose not to have a service and recognize the person in some other way. Your loved one can be included in these decisions.
- Be aware that after the death you may wish to change your mind about some of the details. You are not showing any disrespect if you choose to do that.

DECISIONS AFTER DEATH

What you need to consider
When your loved one dies, there are immediate details that need attention.

Practical details
Several of the following practical aspects of planning may have been decided in advance.
- Inform family members and close friends about the death.
- If flowers and a printed program are to be used, assign someone to arrange for these.

- Write a newspaper obituary. During this stressful time, it is easy to make mistakes with details so be sure someone reads the final copy carefully before submitting it.
- If you wish money given to a charity, you need to decide what this will be. It can be included in the obituary announcement.
- Keep track of cards, visitors and donations so you can acknowledge these at a quieter time.

Planning a Funeral or Memorial Service

If you have planned a service in advance, you may already have decided some of these points. The memorial society or funeral home can guide you on some details.

- A service can take the form of a funeral, a memorial or a simple graveside service.
- Sometimes a bedside service is chosen. If direct cremation has been chosen, this will be the last opportunity for people to see their loved one.
- If you do not have a regular place of worship, you will need to consider where a service will be held. Options include a funeral chapel, a community hall or your home.
- You will need to decide who will officiate at a service. Depending on the form you choose, it may be a religious leader, friend, family member or chaplain.
- You will need to decide if your loved one is to be buried or cremated.
  - If buried, do you already have a plot you wish to use?
  - If cremated, will the remains be buried, kept or scattered?
  - Sometimes after a cremation, people create a "memory place" where the ashes are buried and they can go to visit.
- Some people make an audio or video tape of the service. This way, the carefully chosen words can be replayed anytime, and can be sent to those who could not attend the service. Even family members who attend the funeral often appreciate being able to see or hear it again when they are less upset.
- In any planning you do, consider the schedules of people coming from out of town.

NECESSARY VITAL STATISTICS

The District Registrar of Deaths requires the following information about the person who died. You will need this information when you meet with the funeral director. The funeral director will record and forward it, along with Medical Certificate of Death, to Vital Statistics, Ministry of Health. This information is needed for the funeral director to obtain a permit for burial or cremation and a death certificate.

Name
_____
LAST NAME   ALL GIVEN NAMES

Address
_____
HOUSE/APARTMENT # STREET/ROAD   CITY/TOWN   POSTAL CODE

Marital Status (marriage certificate may be required)
_____
                          SINGLE/MARRIED/WIDOWED/DIVORCED

Maiden Name
_____

Occupation
_____

Birthdate (birth certificate may be required)   Age
_____
                          (MONTH/DAY/YEAR)

Birthplace
_____
CITY/TOWN   PROV/COUNTRY   IF NATIVE, GIVE BAND

Date of Death   Place of Death
_____

Father's Name   Father's Birthplace
_____

Mother's Name   Mother's Maiden Name
_____

Mother's Birthplace
_____

Sex   Height   Weight   Religion
_____

Next of kin
_____
NAME

Address
_____
HOUSE/APARTMENT # STREET/ROAD   CITY/TOWN   POSTAL CODE

Alberta Health Care Number
_____

Family doctor
_____
NAME

Address
_____
HOUSE/APARTMENT # STREET/ROAD   CITY/TOWN

Social Insurance Number
_____

PLACES TO NOTIFY

- Contact the funeral director to complete arrangements.

Funeral director   Phone

- Complete the Vital Statistics Guide and take it to your appointment with the funeral director.
- Contact the Executor/trix or lawyers involved with the will.

Executor/trix   Phone

Co-executor/trix   Phone

Lawyer   Phone

- Prepare a list of people to be notified. Ask someone to help you with the telephoning.

Telephone Helper   Phone

- If desired, write an obituary notice to be printed in the newspaper of your choice. This can be costly so you may want to consider its length, how many insertions, and in which newspapers. The funeral director can assist you with this.

Newspaper   Phone

- If you wish, write or telephone acknowledgement of flowers, cards and donations. Many charitable organizations send thank-you cards to donors and notify the family of any donations received.

Named Charity   Phone

- Notify Canada Pension, banks, landlord or mortgage company, insurance company, utility company, land registry and motor vehicle offices. You will most likely require several copies of the Death Certificate to complete arrangements with them.

Canada Pension Office   Phone

Bank   Phone

Landlord/Mortgage Co.   Phone

Insurance Company   Phone

- Most benefits are not automatic and must be applied for. You should contact:
  - Canada Pension Plan Office - you must apply for benefits (lump sum death benefit, survivor's benefits, dependent children's benefits). You will need your own and the deceased's Social Insurance Numbers.

  Your S.I.N. _____   Deceased S.I.N. _____

- The person's life insurance companies (if relevant)

  Insurance Co. _____   Phone _____

  Insurance Co. _____   Phone _____

- Private Pension Plans

  Pension Plan _____   Phone _____

  Pension Plan _____   Phone _____

- Department of Veterans Affairs - If the person had served in the Canadian Armed Forces, dependents may be eligible for a pension.

  Military I.D. # _____   Phone _____

- Any other memberships that have death benefits e.g. Union, Canadian Automobile Association, Credit Union, fraternal orders.

  Phone _____

  Phone _____

  Phone _____

- Contact medical and health people not immediately involved with the person's death.

a) **Alberta Health Care
    Insurance Commission**

    10025 Jasper Ave
    Box 1360
    Edmonton, AB T5J 2N3
    Phone: Edmonton, 780-427-1432;

    Elsewhere in Alberta,
    call toll-free 310-0000 and ask for 427-1432

b)   **Alberta Blue Cross**

        Phone 780-428-1110

Phone and give: name of deceased, birthdate, date of death, Alberta Health Care Insurance number, dependent's name and birthdate. Dependents must contact these offices within three months to have new cards issued in their own names.

- Contact any clubs, associations, library, magazines, book clubs, etc. of which the person was a member.

_____ Phone _____

_____ Phone _____

_____ Phone _____

_____ Phone _____

_____ Phone _____

_____ Phone _____

- Contact your car insurance agency (if registration is in the person's name, you may need new registration).

_____ Phone _____

_____ Phone _____

GRIEF

When people are trying to adjust to the death of a loved one, they usually grieve. Grief is part of a healing process that helps a person let go of the past and adjust to life without the loved one who has died.

What you need to know

The death of a loved one is followed by clearly understood responses to grief. They may not come in a predictable sequence and they may overlap. Sometimes you may not feel the intensity of your loss until months later. Unfortunately a grieving person does not always realize that the experience is perfectly normal.

- Grief can be hard, stressful and tiring, but it is not an illness.
- Shock and numbness are often the first stages of grief. This is natural even when the death is expected.
- You may feel guilty and have a sense of failure. A period of thinking "if only" is common.
- Anger is a frequent and normal reaction to death. Often it is directed toward the person who died. Sometimes it may be aimed at other people or things unrelated to the death. It can range from mild irritability to rage. If you feel angry, do not try to suppress the feeling. Just accept that this is a natural part of grieving.
- You will probably feel a deep sadness and loneliness after the death of a loved one.
- You may deny the death to protect yourself from the pain of grief.
- Everyone grieves differently. There are no quick fixes or set ways to grieve.
- The pain of loss never goes away but lessens over time.

How grief can affect you physically

You may experience such a wide range of physical symptoms that you begin to think you are ill. These are a physical reaction to your grief. They include:

- tight chest, palpitations
- diarrhea, constipation, vomiting
- lack of energy, weakness
- restlessness
- trouble sleeping or sleeping too much
- decreased sexual drive
- shortness of breath
- crying, sighing
- dizziness, shivering, faintness
- loss of appetite, overeating
- increased alcohol or drug use

How grief can affect you mentally

While you are grieving, your mental state may cause many feelings that you have never experienced before. These include:

- poor concentration
- confusion, "this can't be real"
- constant thoughts about the person
- day dreaming
- nightmares, dreams of loss

How grief can affect you emotionally

In grief, your emotions may change from hour to hour. This is normal and will settle with time. The range of emotions you might experience include:

- shock, numbness, emptiness
- withdrawn or explosive moods
- anger, rage
- denial, disbelief
- frustration
- guilt, regrets
- pining or yearning
- sadness, depression, despair
- loneliness, isolation

How grief can affect you spiritually

No matter what your beliefs, you may go through a period of deep spiritual upheaval. The issues may include:

- blaming life, yourself or the person who has died
- lack of meaning or purpose in life
- wanting to die so you can join the dead person
- continuing to ask "why did this happen?"
- blaming or feeling separation from your spiritual power

How grief can affect you socially

When you are grieving, you may feel as if you are alone in understanding the importance of your loss. You may want the support of others, yet be unwilling to allow them to get close because you believe that no one can appreciate what you are going through. Your feelings may include:

- unrealistic expectations
- lack of interest in others' activities

- withdrawal from others
- dependence on others
- fear of being alone
- feeling out of place with previous friendships
- rushing into new relationships

CHILDREN AND GRIEVING

Children do grieve, but not always like adults. Their understanding, the way they react and what helps them, often varies by age.

- All ages sense the sadness, feel the loss and pain, fear death and being left alone.
- All ages may feel guilt for what has happened.
- Children under three years of age cannot grasp that death is forever.
- Children under 10 years may fear getting sick and dying. If the loved one who died was a parent, a child may worry that the other parent will die too.
- Children over 10 understand better but may not be able to talk about death.

How you can offer comfort and care to children

How parents grieve affects the way their children grieve. People who smile bravely when they are sad confuse children. Adults who admit their feelings and cry with their children help them to accept and understand death. Some books that might help children during their grief are suggested on page 126.

- Include the child in what is happening.
- Tell the truth and give lots of support.
- Listen carefully to the meaning behind what children are saying about their feelings.
- Be honest and give answers in words they understand.
- Reassure children that illness does not always lead to death.
- Remind children that they are loved just as much as ever during your time of grief.
- Tell children that their thoughts and feelings are normal and it is okay to cry.
- Reassure them that others understand their grief.
- Encourage them to express feelings by talking, painting, poetry, puppets and music.
- Try to keep the children's routine as much the same as possible.

TAKING CARE OF YOURSELF WHEN GRIEVING

It is difficult to anticipate how you will react when death occurs. The important thing to remember is that there are no right or wrong ways to behave. Do whatever feels right.

- Accept your need to grieve and to feel your loss. It is okay to cry and express your sadness.
- Talk about your feelings if this gives you comfort. Choose someone you are comfortable with who is a good listener.
- Take your time in resuming your regular activities. Be patient with yourself when you are confused or forgetful.
- Look after yourself physically. Eat well, exercise and get lots of rest. Poor nutrition leaves you at risk of health problems. Do something nice for yourself each day.
- Explore what life and death mean to you.
- Do not isolate yourself. Meet with old friends, talk about your loss, mention your loved one by name.
- Be careful when driving. Poor concentration and 'blanking out' can be hazardous.
- Slow down and let some responsibilities go for a time. Low energy is to be expected.
- Restrict drugs and alcohol. They can depress your ability to think clearly.
- Recognize that palpitations, digestive problems, chest pains, shortness of breath are all normal reactions to grief, but it is important to contact your doctor and have them checked out anyway.
- Make time to do the things you enjoy and just go on living.
- Try to focus on positive things each day.
- Take time to be alone when you need it.
- If prayer is a part of your normal life, be gentle with yourself if it takes a while before you start to pray again. Let others continue to carry you in their prayers.
- See the resources listed on page 123 for suggestions that you and your loved ones might find helpful during this time of grief.

HOW LONG GRIEF MAY LAST

It is hard to say how long a person will experience intense grief. People mistakenly think you should be "back to normal" in three months but this is not the case.

- Many people find that grief comes and goes in waves for a long time.
- After several months intense feelings begin to ease.
- It may take many months, or even longer, before you feel more balanced, have new interests and find that life slowly begins to have meaning again.
- Over time coping gets easier and confidence begins to return.
- It may take you a long time to return to places or things you used to enjoy together before the death.
- Although you may develop a new and full life, it may take years to feel you can exist fully without the person who died.
- Even when you think you are over your grief, feelings may be triggered by memories, places, songs, films or poems.
- Feelings of grief ease and become part of your life.

IMPORTANT POINTS

You need to find ways to cope. Ask yourself what has helped in facing past difficulties, and use those methods now. If or when these no longer help, be honest with yourself when you answer the following questions.
Since the death are you:

- always bad tempered and angry?
- busy all the time, restless or unable to keep your mind on what you should be doing?
- afraid of getting too close to other people for fear of facing loss again?
- finding that you keep going over and over the same things in your mind?
- unable to get rid of guilt about what you did or did not do before the person died?
- feeling all the time as if you are numb and alone?
- often thinking about your own death?
- doing things that may prove harmful to yourself such as drinking a lot of liquor, using more medications, driving without care?
- having frequent thoughts of suicide?
- more fearful for no good reason?

Grief can pass over into a clinical depression that may need professional help. If you answer yes to any of the above questions more than one year after the death, see your doctor for help.

FINAL THOUGHTS

For some people, much of the grief was experienced before the death. The death itself brings a sense of closure and healing has already begun. For others, the process of grief may take longer. For everyone, healing can take many forms as life gradually returns to normal.

- There may be a tremendous sense of relief that the suffering of the person is over.
- As you have time to reflect, you may develop intense pride in the courage and dignity shown by the person who was dying.
- You may feel a strong bond with family and friends who have supported you.
- Happiness with the pleasures of life may begin to return.
- There may be a sense of a new start in life with new experiences.
- You may want to live life to the fullest to make up for the fact that your loved one will not have the opportunity.

You will always remember the person who died. That person played an important part in your life so keep the memories alive in your heart and mind. Take comfort in knowing that by giving care in the final stages of life, you shared in the most loving act of support and comfort.

Books and other resources that may be helpful

WRITTEN MATERIALS

Albom, Mitch. (1997). *Tuesdays with Morrie: An old man, a young man and the last great lesson.* Toronto: Doubleday Canada, Limited.

Berry, L. & Schneider, T. (1997). *What do I do now?* Red Deer, AB: Eventide Funeral Chapels. [Pamphlet: to obtain, contact Eventide Funeral Chapels in Red Deer, AB (403) 347-2222.]

Buckman, R. (1988). *I don't know what to say.* Toronto, ON: Key Porter Books Limited.

Byock, I. (1997). *Dying well.* New York, NY: Riverhead Books.

Callanan, M. & Kelley, P. (1997). *Final gifts: Understanding the special awareness, needs, and communications of the dying.* Bantam Books Canada, Incorporated.

Canadian Cancer Society. (1985). *Taking time: Support for people living with cancer and people who care about them.* Bethesda, MD: National Cancer Institute. [Pamphlet: to obtain contact Canadian Cancer Society.]

Canadian Cancer Society. (1983). *Nutrition for people with cancer.* Toronto, ON: Department of Nutrition at the Ontario Cancer Institute, Princess Margaret Hospital and the Canadian Cancer Society.

Deachman, M., & Howell, D. (1991). *Supportive care at home: A guide for terminally ill patients and their families.* Markham, ON: Knoll Pharmaceuticals Canada [Pamphlet: to obtain contact Knoll Pharmaceuticals Canada, Markham, ON.]

Golden, S. (1988). *Nursing a loved one at home: A care giver's guide.* Philadelphia, PA: Running Press.

Grollman, E. A. (1987). *In sickness and in health: how to cope when your loved one is ill.* Boston: Beacon Press.

Grollman, E. A. (1993). *Straight talk about death for teenagers: how to cope with losing someone you love.* Boston: Beacon Press.

Grollman, E. A. (1976). *Talking about death: a dialogue between parent and child.* Boston: Beacon Press.

Jevne, R. F. (1994). *The voice of hope: heard across the heart of life.* San Diego, CA: Lura Media.

Jevne, R. F. (1991). *It all begins with hope: patients, caregivers & the bereaved speak out.* San Diego, CA: Lura Media.

Jevne, R. F., & Levitan, A. (1989). *No time for nonsense: self-help for the seriously ill.* San Diego, CA: Lura Media.

Kübler-Ross, E. (1970). *On death and dying.* New York: Macmillan.

Kübler-Ross, E. (1981). *On children and death.* New York: Collier Books.

Kübler-Ross, E. (1983). *Living with death and dying.* New York: Macmillan.

Latimer, E. J. (1996). *Easing the hurt: A handbook of comfort for families and friends of people who are seriously ill.* Hamilton, ON: Purdue Frederick. [Pamphlet: to obtain contact Purdue Frederick Inc., 575 Granite Court, Pickering, Ontario, L1W 3W8.]

McFarlane, R., & Bashe, P. (1998). *The complete bedside companion: A no-nonsense guide to caring for the seriously ill.* New York: Simon & Schuster.

Mertick, E. (1991). Yours, mine and our children's grief: A parent's guide. Calgary, AB: Alberta Funeral Service Association. [Pamphlet: to obtain contact Alberta Funeral Service Association, 1-800-803-8809.]

Paulus, Trina. (1973/1997). *Hope for the Flowers.* New Jersey: Paulist Press.

Rando, T. A. (1991). *How to go on living when someone you love dies.* New York: Bantam Books.

Siegel, B. S. (1990). *Love, medicine & miracles: Lessons learned about self-healing from a surgeon's experience with exceptional.* New York: Harper Perennial.

Siegel, B. S. (1989). *Peace, love & healing: body mind communication and the path to self-healing: An exploration.* New York: Harper & Row.

van Bommel, H. (1999). *Caring for loved ones at home.* Scarborough, ON: Resources Supporting Family and Community Legacies Inc. [Book: to obtain contact Resources Supporting Family and Community Legacies Inc. (416) 264-4665.]

White, P. (Ed.). (1986). *Home care of the hospice patient: An informational/instructional booklet for caregivers in the home.* Chicago, IL: Rush-Presbyterian-St. Luke's Medical Centre. [Pamphlet: to obtain contact Purdue Frederick Inc., 575 Granite Court Pickering, Ontario, L1W 3W8.]

BOOKS TO HELP GRIEVING CHILDREN

Buscaglia, L. (1983). *The fall of Freddie the leaf.* Holt, Rinehart & Winston. [A story that uses nature and the changing seasons of life to explain how death can be seen as a natural part of living. Hardcover, ages 4 - 8, 36 pages.]

Gobie, P. (1993). *Beyond the ridge.* Aladdin Paperbacks. [This is a Native American story that gives a beautiful introduction to a way of seeing death as a spiritual pathway leading into a new life - a life filled with beauty, peace and love. Paperback, ages 4 - 8, 32 pages.]

Gootman, M., Espeland, P, & Prothrow-Smith, D. (1994). *When a friend dies.* Free Spirit Publishers. [This book guides teens with gentle advice after the death of a friend. Paperback, young adult, 108 pages.]

Grollman, E. (1993). *Straight talk about death.* Beacon Press. [Written by a rabbi who offers information about the thoughts, feelings and questions a teenager might have when a loved one dies. Paperback, young adult, 146 pages.]

Grollman, E. (1991). *Talking about death.* Beacon Press. [A book to help adults explain death to young children. It has illustrated stories and sensitive advice to comfort and educate children; paperback, 118 pages.]

Krementz, J. (1998). *How it feels when a parent dies.* Knopf. [A book combining photographs and the personal stories of 18 young people ages 7 - 16 who come from a variety of cultural, social and economic backgrounds. They speak of their feelings and difficulties, and eventual overcoming of grief after the death of a parent. Paperback, all ages, 112 pages.]

Potok, C. (1998). *Zebra and other stories.* Knopf. [Six stories in which young people face crisis or grief and see themselves, their parents and the world around them in a new light. They are stories that build hope. Hardcover, young adults, 146 pages.]

Traisman, E. S. (1992). *Fire in my heart, ice in my veins.* Centering Corp. [A journal for teenagers where they can record thoughts, feelings and questions related to the death of a loved one. Each page provides a brief thought-starter as a focus for writing. Paperback, young adult, 70 pages.]

Vigna, J. & Levine, A. (1991). *Saying goodbye to daddy.* Albert Whitman & Co. [This is a story about a girl who is angry, lonely and frightened after her father is killed in a car accident. She is lovingly cared for and helped by her mother and grandmother. Hardcover, ages 4 - 8, 36 pages.]

INTERNET RESOURCES

Capital Health Regional Palliative Care Program, Patients and Family, Section [www.palliative.org/patient_family.html]

Caregiver Network (Canadian) [www.caregiver.on.ca:80/index]

Caregiver Survival Resources (American) [www.caregiver911.com]

Death NET (American) [www.rights.org/~deathnet/open.html]

Dying Well (American) [http://dyingwell.com]

Eldercare Web (American) [//www.elderweb.com/index.shtml]

Glaxo–Wellcome Foundation and Canadian Palliative Care Association (Canadian) *Living Lessons* [www.livinglessons.org]

Hopewell House. (1999). Guide through the journey of dying [www.hospiceweb.com/states/oregon/hopewell/journey.htm]

Hospice Net, For Patients and Families Facing Life-Threatening Illness [www.hospicenet.org]

Living with Grief - When a loved one is dying [www.caregivertips.com]

Mount, B. M. (1999). The ACP home care guide for advanced cancer. American College of Physicians [www.acponline.org/public/h_care/contents.htm]

van Bommel, H. (1998). Family Hospice Care [http://Home.InfoRamp.Net/~harryvb/books/hospicecare/toc.htm]

REFERENCES USED IN PREPARATION OF THIS BOOK

Berry, L. & Schneider, T. (1997). *What do I do now?* Red Deer, AB: Eventide Funeral Chapels.

Buckman, R. (1988). *I don't know what to say.* Toronto, ON: Key Porter Books Limited.

Canadian Cancer Society. (1983). *Nutrition for people with cancer.* Toronto, ON: Department of Nutrition at the Ontario Cancer Institute, Princess Margaret Hospital and the Canadian Cancer Society.

Canadian Cancer Society. (1985). *Taking time: Support for people living with cancer and people who care about them.* Bethesda, MD: National Cancer Institute.

Canadian Palliative Care Association and the Canadian Association for Community Care. (1998). *Training manual for support workers in palliative care.* Ottawa, ON: Canadian Palliative Care Association.

Cantwell, P., MacKay, S., Macmillan, K., Turco, S., McKinnon, S., Read-Paul, L. (1988). *99 common questions (and answers) about palliative care: a nurse's handbook.* Edmonton, AB: Regional Palliative Care Program, Capital Health Authority.

Capital Health Home Care (1996) *Changing your Infusion Tubing* and *Preloading a single insulin.*

Cassileth, B. R. (Ed.). (1986). *Caring for the terminally ill patient at home: A guide for family caregivers.* University of Pennsylvania Cancer Centre Hospice and Homecare Program.

Deachman, M., & Howell, D. (1991). *Supportive care at home: A guide for terminally ill patients and their families.* Markham, ON: Knoll Pharmaceuticals Canada.

Ferris, F. D., Flannery, J. S., McNeal, H. B., Morissette, M. R., Cameron, R., & Bally, G. A. (1995). *Module 4: Palliative Care. A comprehensive guide for the care of persons with HIV disease.* Toronto, ON: Mount Sinai Hospital and Casey House Hospice.

Hopewell House. (1999). *Guide through the journey of dying.* [Online]. Available: www.hospiceweb.com/states/oregon/hopewell/journey.htm

Jones, C. M., & Pegis, J. (1994). *The palliative patient: Principles of treatment.* Markham, ON: Knoll Pharma Inc.

Latimer, E. J. (1996). *Easing the hurt: A handbook of comfort for families and friends of people who are seriously ill.* Hamilton, ON: Purdue Frederick.

Mertick, E. (1991). *Yours, mine and our children's grief: A parent's guide.* Calgary, AB: Alberta Funeral Service Association.

Mount, B. M. (1999). *The ACP home care guide for advanced cancer.* American College of Physicians. [Online]. Available: www.acponline.org/public/h_care/contents.htm

Pereira, J., & Bruera, E. (1997). *The Edmonton aid to palliative care.* Edmonton, AB: Division of Palliative Care, University of Alberta.

White, P. (1986). *Home care of the hospice patient: An informational/ instructional booklet for caregivers in the home.* Chicago, IL: Rush-Presbyterian-St. Luke's Medical Centre.

van Bommel, H. (1999). *Caring for loved ones at home.* Scarborough, ON: Saint Elizabeth Health Care Foundation; Resources Supporting Family and Community Legacies Inc.

Victoria Hospice Society. (1993). *Palliative care at home.* Volume II. Victoria, BC: Victoria Hospice Society.

Victoria Hospice Society. (1995). *Palliative care for home support workers.* Volume III. Victoria, BC: Victoria Hospice Society.

FINANCIAL AID

There are many resources available that may help you financially while you are caring for your loved one who is terminally ill. Ask a member of your health care team for advice about the following possibilities or if there is other assistance in your community.

Canada Pension Plan

A disability pension is payable to anyone under 65 who has contributed to the Canada Pension Plan for a specified period of time, and has a severe and prolonged disability.

Phone: 1-800-661-3921

Guaranteed Income Supplement

You may be eligible for this supplement, if you are over 65 and depending on your income. For example, if your only income is the Old Age Security, you would most likely qualify.

Phone: 1-800-277-9914

Old Age Security

If you or the person you are caring for turns 65 during this period of palliative care, be aware the Old Age Security will not come automatically. An application should be submitted six months before the 65th birthday and you may need to help begin this process.

Phone: 1-800-277-9914

Social Assistance

If you receive social assistance, you may qualify for financial help with medical expenses, prescriptions and special health needs. If you do not already receive social assistance, but do have a low income, you may also be able to get help with certain expenses. The phone number of the office closest to your home will be listed in the phone book under Government of Alberta, Human Resources and Employment or:

Phone: Edmonton, 780-427-2734
             Calgary, 403-297-4575

Elsewhere in Alberta, toll-free, 310-0000
and ask for one of the above numbers.

Employment Insurance

You qualify for Employment Insurance if you have made contributions for 20 of the last 52 weeks.

Phone: 1-800-206-7218

Department of Veterans Affairs (DVA)

If your loved one is a veteran, you may be eligible for:
- an attendance allowance for care given during the illness.
- a disability pension.
- equipment and home alternations.

Contact a DVA counsellor to discuss your situation. You will need to know the person's service number.

Phone: 1-800-866-1240

Private Insurance Plan

Check the extended health plan from an employer. Benefits covered may include ambulance, nursing care, Home Support Aide, medications, oxygen.

Alberta Palliative Care Drug Coverage

This program subsidizes the cost of some medications used by a person receiving palliative care at home. A doctor must confirm on an application that palliative care is being given. When the application is accepted, the required medications can be obtained at your local pharmacy. Full details are available from Alberta Health and Wellness.

Phone: Edmonton, 780-422-0102
              Calgary, 403-297-6411

Elsewhere in Alberta, toll-free: 310-0000
and ask for one of the above numbers.

Life Insurance Policies

If a family member has a serious illness, it may be possible to apply to have your premiums waived without affecting the policy itself. This requires a written application and medical proof of illness.

Associations, Lodges and Unions

Check with lodges or other organizations to which the person belongs to see if they provide financial help during a member's illness.

Canadian Cancer Society

This group provides financial help with certain medications. There is also assistance with transportation and accommodation. There is a means test to determine eligibility for this program. Call the number listed in your telephone book or

Phone: 1-888-939-3333

Revenue Canada

When a person has been disabled for an extended time, there may be income tax deducations for that person, dependents and medical expenses.

Phone: 1-800-661-4597

Assured Income for the Severely Handicapped (AISH)

The AISH program provides financial help to adults with severe and permanent disabilities. The amount of money people receive depends on their income. AISH is not a medical program. People receive AISH if their disability is permanent, meaning they have exhausted all opportunities for rehabilitation, training and work. For more information regarding AISH, contact Alberta Family & Social Services.

Phone: Edmonton, 780-415-6300
            Calgary, 403-297-8511

Elsewhere in Alberta, toll-free: 310-0000
and ask for one of the above numbers.

Last Post Fund

If your loved one left no money and/or was on a war pension, and was a veteran of World War I or II or the Korean Campaign, burial costs may be covered by the Last Post Fund. Any branch of the Royal Canadian Legion (ask for the Service Officer) or the Department of Veterans Affairs can assist you, or the Funeral Director will complete the application for you if you supply the regimental number. Contact the following before funeral arrangements are made.

Phone: Edmonton, 780-495-3766, Fax: 780-495-6960
            Calgary, 403-244-6821, Fax: 403-270-8555

Special Needs Assistance for Seniors

This is an Alberta government grant program that provides financial assistance to low income seniors who are experiencing financial difficulties.

Phone: Edmonton, 780-2585

Elsewhere in Alberta, toll-free, 1-800-642-3853

LEGAL AFFAIRS

Sometimes it is necessary for one person to act on behalf of another. Three categories of legally binding documents allow the care of an incapacitated person. These documents are power of attorney, guardianship and trusteeship. A fourth category is a personal directive. This is not legally binding but is a statement of a person's wishes.

Enduring Power of Attorney

An enduring power of attorney is a document that appoints a person to act financially on behalf of someone else who is either physically or mentally incapacitated. A power of attorney should be prepared far in advance of being needed as a safeguard. It is obtained through a lawyer. The person giving the permission must be of sound mind, alert and able to make decisions. Otherwise the person acting on the power of attorney order is acting without authority. The advantage of the power of attorney is that it gives a dying person the chance to decide who will be managing financial affairs.

Guardianship

This order is granted by the courts under the Dependent Adults Act. When a person is not able to make decisions such as where to live, health care and daily needs, guardianship permits another person to make these decisions. The guardian is required to decide in the best interest of the person, to encourage independence and to act in the least restrictive manner possible.

Trusteeship

This is an order under the Dependent Adults Act that gives a person permission to handle the financial affairs of another. The trustee can assume control when someone's mental condition prevents sound decision-making. Legal authority is given to manage, handle, administer, sell and dispose of assets just as the person could have done. Restrictions may be imposed by the judge and the trustee must file a full inventory and account of assets and liabilities.

A Trustee and a Guardian may both be needed for the same person if the ability to make decisions about daily living and about finances is impaired. To obtain a Trustee or Guardianship order, the assistance of a solicitor is required and a medical report must be filed with the court.

Old Age Security Trusteeship

This type of trusteeship is for handling cheques for someone else. It allows an appointed person to cash or deposit cheques for another. Cheques may not be written on the account nor funds withdrawn.

Personal Directive

A personal directive states a person's wishes about medical care if that person is not able to make the decisions. While it is not a legal document, it is intended to ensure that the individual's rights are honoured. Details of a personal directive need to be discussed fully with both your family doctor and immediate family members.

The Alberta government has produced several pamphlets to help you write this document. Contact the Office of the Public Guardian at the numbers below to request free copies. There is also detailed information on the Alberta Health and Wellness Web site at: www.health.gov.ab.ca/public/document/pdguide.htm.

For further information about the above topics, ask a member of your health care team or contact:

The Office of the Public Guardian
Edmonton: 780-427-7945
Calgary: 403-297-6251

Elsewhere in Alberta, toll-free: 310-0000
and ask for one of the above numbers.

HOME MEDICATION SCHEDULE

															Date
															Name of Medication
															Dose
															How Taken
															Purpose
															12 MIDNIGHT
															2 am
															4 am
															6 am
															8 am
															10 am
															12 NOON
															2 pm
															4 pm
															6 pm
															8 pm
															10 pm

This page may be photocopied.

SYMPTOM ASSESSMENT SCALE

Circle the number that best describes:

No Pain	0 1 2 3 4 5 6 7 8 9 10	Worst Possible Pain
Not Tired	0 1 2 3 4 5 6 7 8 9 10	Worst Possible Tiredness
Not Nauseated	0 1 2 3 4 5 6 7 8 9 10	Worst Possible Nausea
Not Depressed	0 1 2 3 4 5 6 7 8 9 10	Worst Possible Depression
Not Drowsy	0 1 2 3 4 5 6 7 8 9 10	Worst Possible Drowsiness
Not Anxious	0 1 2 3 4 5 6 7 8 9 10	Worst Possible Anxiety
Best Appetite	0 1 2 3 4 5 6 7 8 9 10	Worst Possible Appetite
Best Feeling of Wellbeing	0 1 2 3 4 5 6 7 8 9 10	Worst Possible feeling of Wellbeing
No Shortness of Breath	0 1 2 3 4 5 6 7 8 9 10	Worst Possible Shortness of Breath
Other Problem	0 1 2 3 4 5 6 7 8 9 10	

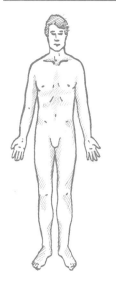 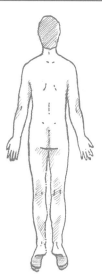

Mark on these pictures where it is that you hurt.

BREAK THROUGH MEDICATION CHART

Date	Medication	Dose	How Taken	Initial	Time Given (write time in box)

Write in when the Break Through Analgesic (BTA) was given.

This page may be photocopied.

INSERTING AND REMOVING A SUBCUTANEOUS NEEDLE

INSERTING A SUBCUTANEOUS NEEDLE

The following is an outline of how to start a subcutaneous needle and use it to give medications. It can serve as a reminder after you have been taught by your home care nurse. You should never attempt any procedure unless you are certain you know how to do it correctly. If in doubt, wait for help from your home care nurse.

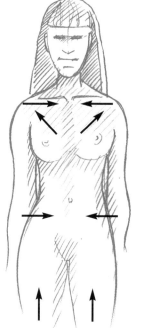

figure 28

- Explain the reason for the subcutaneous needle and reassure the person.
- Gather the equipment you need:
  - winged needle (25 G)
  - tape
  - transparent dressing or band aid or tape only
  - 70% isopropyl alcohol swab or 0.5% chlorhexidine (in case of allergy to alcohol or chlorhexidine use povidone iodine)
  - non-sterile gloves if contact with blood should be avoided (such as HIV infection).
- Before you begin, explain to the person what you will be doing.
- Wash your hands. Put on non-sterile gloves if you are using them.
- Ask the person to choose if there is a site preference and the direction the needle should be placed. Be aware of how the needle placement may effect the person's ability to move freely.
- Choose the site. Suggested sites include upper chest (avoiding breast tissue), below the shoulder blade, stomach and thigh (do not use thigh if the person is active). The upper chest is most commonly used.
- Choose the direction of the needle. (See figures 28 and 29)
  - In the abdomen, direct the needle across the abdomen to stop pinching or grabbing when the person sits or bends.
  - In the chest, the needle may be placed in any direction. Avoid breast tissue as the solution may stay in one spot in this area, and not be effective.
  - Do not put the needle in the arm pit because the solution will not be absorbed as well and the needle will be uncomfortable.

- Clean the site with 70% isopropyl alcohol swab or 0.5% chlorhexidine swab. Move in a circular motion from the centre of where you are going to put the needle. Allow
the area to dry for 30 seconds.
- Insert winged needle. (See figure 30)
  - Gently pinch a generous amount of tissue between your index finger and thumb.
    - Insert needle at a 45-degree angle into the fold of tissue you are holding, bevel side up.
- Cover the insertion site with a bandaid or transparent dressing over the wings of the needle and the site. The importance of this is to keep the needle secure so it cannot move within the vein. (See figure 31a)

  or
- Apply tape to the wing needle using an "H" configuration. (See figure 31b)
- Coil the tubing and secure it with tape to the dressing or skin. (See figure 31c)
- Look at the end of the needle's tubing. If there is a rubber end on the tubing you are ready to given an injection. If there is a plastic cap on the end you will need to put on a cap with a rubber end (Heparin Lok™) to given injections into the site. (See figure 31d)
- Once the needle is inserted there should be no further discomfort.

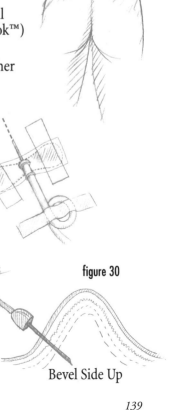

figure 29

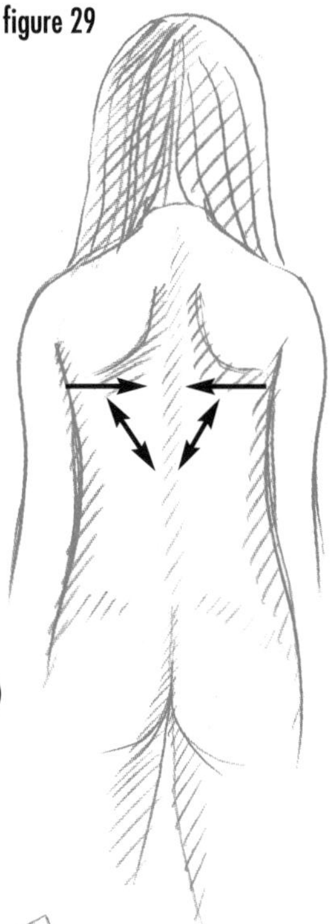

figure 31b

figure 31a

figure 31c

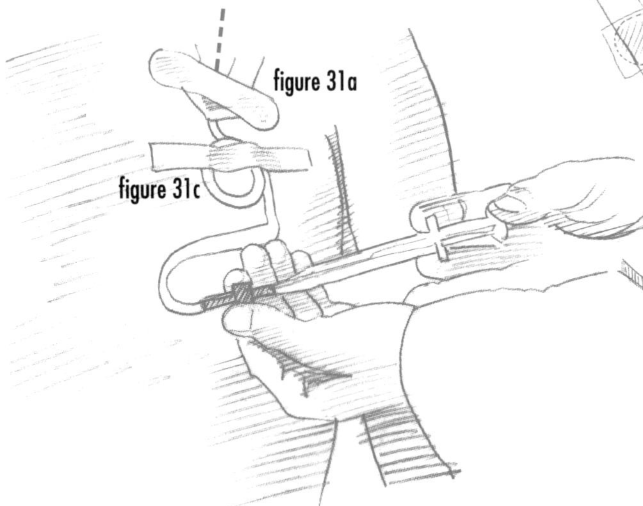

figure 30

Bevel Side Up

REMOVING A SUBCUTANEOUS NEEDLE

- Remove all the tape and the dressing where the needle goes in with one hand while holding the needle in place with the other.
- Pinch the wings of the butterfly needle up between your index finger and thumb and pull the needle out.
- Hold a piece of gauze on the site briefly to stop any fluid that leaks.
- Dispose of the needle properly in a container that is puncture proof and has a lid (see Infection Control, p.26).

PREPARING THE MEDICATION

With a subcutaneous needle in place, you are ready to give a medications into the cap at the end of the needle's tubing.

What you need to know

Talk with your pharmacist or home care nurse about how the medication will be provided. Some of them will preload the medication into syringes for you.

- If different doses of the medication are needed the nurse or pharmacist may teach you how to draw up the medication into the syringe. If you are given the syringe with the medication already drawn up, skip to the section on how to give the injection.
- Wash your hands.
- Gather the equipment you will need:
  - ampule or vial of medication
  - syringe and needle
  - alcohol swab
  - container to put needle and glass in after use
- An ampule is a small glass container with a pointed top and is intended for only one dose of the medication.
  - Tap the top of the ampule with a light flick of your finger to make sure all the medication is in the bottom. (See figure 32)
  - Wrap the top of the ampule at the "neck" with the alcohol swab package.

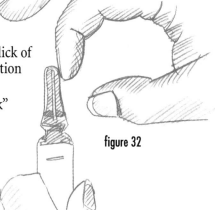

figure 32

- Snap the neck of the ampule quickly away from you. This will break it open. (See figure 33)
- Place the top of the ampule in your disposal container. (Keep the alcohol swab package).
- Remove the cap on the needle of the syringe. Be careful not to touch the needle.

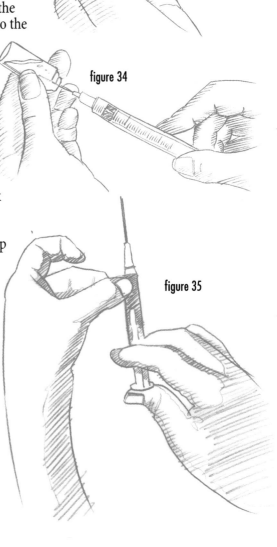

figure 33

- Hold the ampule in your non-dominant hand upside down at a slight angle. Do not worry, the medication will stay in the ampule.
- Put the needle into the centre of the ampule. Draw the medication into the syringe by slowly pulling back on the plunger of the syringe. (See figure 34)

figure 34

- Hold the syringe with the needle pointing to the ceiling, again being careful not to touch the needle.
- Put the ampule into your disposal container.
- Flick the syringe with your index finger to get all the air bubbles in the syringe to the top. Slowly press up on the syringe plunger to get rid of the bubbles. (See figure 35)

figure 35

- Look at the black markings and numbers on the syringe. Slowly push the plunger of the syringe upwards until you have the right dose for the person. Your pharmacist or home care nurse will tell you the right dose of medication.
- You are now ready to give the medication to the person. (Skip the section on vials and go to giving the injection.)

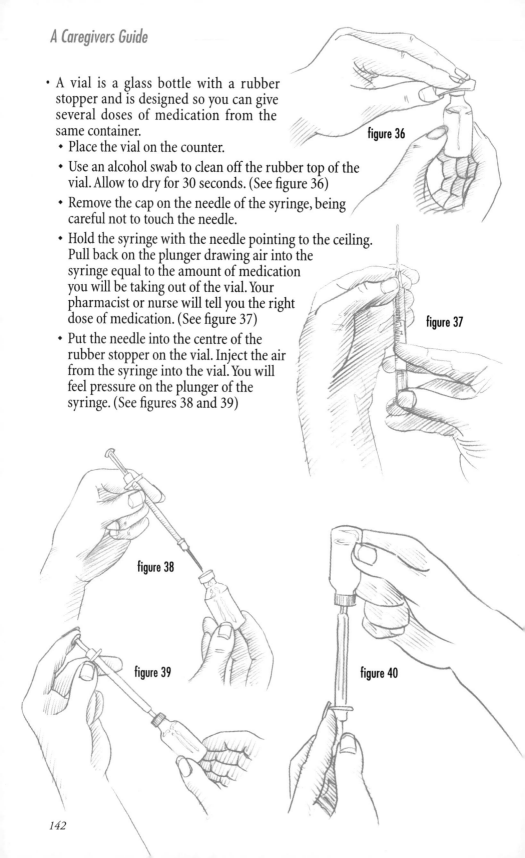

- A vial is a glass bottle with a rubber stopper and is designed so you can give several doses of medication from the same container.
  - Place the vial on the counter.
  - Use an alcohol swab to clean off the rubber top of the vial. Allow to dry for 30 seconds. (See figure 36)
  - Remove the cap on the needle of the syringe, being careful not to touch the needle.
  - Hold the syringe with the needle pointing to the ceiling. Pull back on the plunger drawing air into the syringe equal to the amount of medication you will be taking out of the vial. Your pharmacist or nurse will tell you the right dose of medication. (See figure 37)
  - Put the needle into the centre of the rubber stopper on the vial. Inject the air from the syringe into the vial. You will feel pressure on the plunger of the syringe. (See figures 38 and 39)

figure 36

figure 37

figure 38

figure 39

figure 40

- Turn the vial, with the needle in it, upside down. (See figure 40)
- Pull the needle part way back until it is below the fluid level in the vial.
- Look at the black markings and numbers on the syringe. Gently pull back on the syringe plunger until you have a little more than the right dose of medication in your syringe. This allows for any air that may get into the syringe. Remove the needle from the vial.
- Gently flick the syringe with your finger to get all the air bubbles in the syringe to the top. Slowly press up on the syringe plunger to get rid of the air bubbles and keep pushing until you have the right dose for the person. (See figure 41)

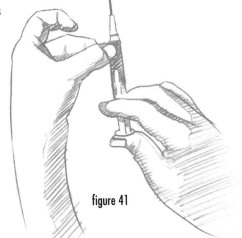

figure 41

- Remember that the vial can be reused. After you have given the injection, store the vial according to the pharmacist's instructions.

GIVING THE INJECTION

If you give the injection slowly through the rubber stopper the person should not have discomfort. Some medications can sting a bit and slowing down the injection may help.

- Clean the rubber injection cap on the person's subcutaneous needle with an alcohol swab. Allow to dry for 30 seconds.
- Stick the syringe needle into the centre of the injection cap. Gently push on the plunger of the syringe, injecting the medication into the person. (See figure 42)

figure 42

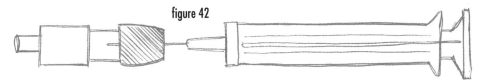

- When all the medication is given, remove the syringe and needle.
- Put the used syringe and needle into your disposal container.
- Store the vial according to your pharmacist's instructions.

STARTING A HYPODERMOCLYSIS

A hypodermoclysis is given through a subcutaneous needle. The procedure for insertion of the needle is the same as described in the section above.

- The doctor will order the type of solution and the pharmacist will make it up. (A solution given this way is called an infusion.)
- Gather the equipment you will need:
  - solution
  - IV tubing
  - IV pole or something to hang the solution bag on

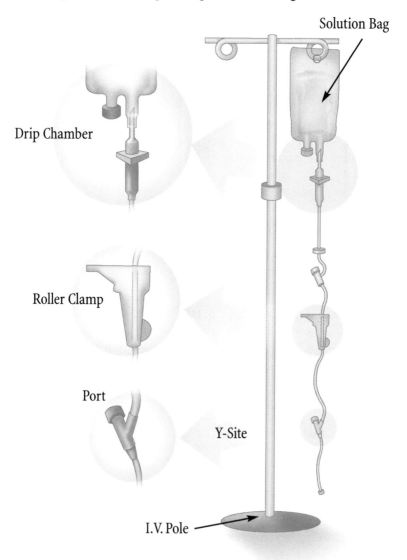

Solution Bag

Drip Chamber

Roller Clamp

Port

Y-Site

I.V. Pole

- Check where the subcutaneous needle is inserted for:
  - redness • pain • bruising
  - swelling • leaking
- Tell your home care nurse if any of the above happens.
- Open the infusion set package.
- Move the roller clamp up the tubing close to the drip chamber (the clear bulge near the top of the tubing). Roll the roller down so that it squeezes the tubing.
- Remove the protective covers from the solution bag and tubing spike. Be careful not to touch the opening.
- Put the spike into the opening in the solution bag.
- Hang the solution on an IV pole. Alternatively you may use a hook in the ceiling or on the wall or any other device that keeps the solution bag higher than the person. This allows the solution to infuse with the help of gravity.
- Squeeze the drip chamber so the solution from the bag drips into it. The drip chamber should only be half full of solution. If the chamber overfills take the solution bag off the pole and squeeze some of the solution in the drip chamber back into the bag.
- Hold the end of the tubing over a glass. Remove the protective end of the tubing, again being careful not to touch the end. Place the protective cap down on a clean surface. (You will need to use the cap again).
- Roll the roller clamp upwards. This will stop the clamp from squeezing the tubing. The solution will flow through the tubing and drip out of the end.
- Roll the roller clamp back down to squeeze the tubing, once the solution is dripping out of the end.
- Put the protective cap back on the end of the tubing.
- Place the tubing end close to the person's subcutaneous site.
- Remove the protective cap from the person's subcutaneous needle tubing being careful not to touch the end of the tubing. Put the cap on a clean surface.
- Remove the protective cap from the solution tubing. Be careful not to touch the end. Place the protective cap on a clean surface.
- Connect the end of the solution tubing and the tubing of the subcutaneous needle tubing. Screw gently together.
- Unroll the roller clamp and adjust how fast the solution is flowing by adjusting the clamp. Your home care nurse will tell you how many drips of solution in the drip chamber is needed in one minute.
- Connect the two protective caps together and put in a safe, clean place.

ONCE THE HYPODERMOCLYSIS IS COMPLETE

The tubing needs to be disconnected when the hypodermoclysis is finished.

- Roll the roller clamp down into the off position.
- Disconnect the two protective caps.
- Disconnect the solution tubing from the subcutaneous needle tubing. Be careful not to touch the endings. Ask the person to hold one of the tubes for you if possible.
- Put the protective caps back on the solution tubing and the subcutaneous needle tubing. By putting the protective caps back on you will stop bacteria from getting into the tubing.
- Leave the bag of solution connected to the IV tubing until the next bag is ready to be infused.
- You can use the same IV tubing for seven days. After seven days a new infusion set will need to be used.
- The subcutaneous needle can stay in place until it needs to be changed because of redness, pain, swelling, bruising or leaking around the needle. Your home care nurse will change it or you can if you have been taught how.

THE PALLIATIVE CARE ASSOCIATION OF ALBERTA

The Palliative Care Association of Alberta (PCAA) is a provincial network consisting of membership from the disciplines of medicine, nursing, social work, pharmacy, pastoral care, rehabilitation and volunteers. The mission of PCAA is to provide leadership and support for end of life care. Since its inception in 1990, PCAA has worked at fostering the growth and development of quality palliative care throughout all parts of Alberta. Earlier initiatives include working with the provincial government to develop the Alberta Health Policy Framework for Palliative Care (1993). PCAA participates in the national forum on palliative care through representation to the Canadian Palliative Care Association. PCAA continues to collaborate with other groups who are committed to enhancement of end of life care.

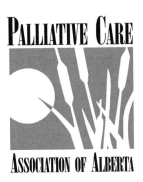

THE MILITARY AND HOSPITALLER ORDER OF ST. LAZARUS OF JERUSALEM

The Military and Hospitaller Order of St. Lazarus of Jerusalem is an international order of chivalry which dates back 900 years to the first Crusades. Since its inception, the Order has been involved with the relief of leprosy both in the Holy Land during the time of the crusades and for several hundred years as a leader in the fight against leprosy in Europe. Still today, the Order supports programs internationally that alleviate the suffering of persons with leprosy. In Canada, the focus of the Order is directed towards palliative care.

The Order of St. Lazarus in Canada, with a membership of approximately 550, is a bilingual, multi-denominational Christian, charitable organization whose goals are to:

- Alleviate the suffering of persons with leprosy
- Care for the aged, sick and needy
- Support medical research
- Promote ecumenism
- Promote national unity and the qualities of good citizenship

Across the country, there are eleven branches known as commanderies: Acadia (Atlantic Canada), Québec, Montréal, Ottawa, Toronto, Western Ontario, Thunder Bay, Manitoba, Edmonton, Calgary and British Columbia.

Recognizing the need to alleviate suffering is a worldwide mission, the Grand Priory of Canada has given assistance to a number of major international projects, including:

- Little Flower Hospital in Bihar, India, is a treatment centre for persons suffering from leprosy partially supported by an annual donation.
- McKean Rehabilitation Centre near Chiang Mai, Thailand, built a special care ward for leprosy patients with money donated by the Order which also provides ongoing support.
- Naini Hospital in Uttar Pradesh, India, a ward for leprosy patients was funded by the Order which continues to support operations with an annual donation.

In accordance with its goals the Order has contributed **to and supported various** organizations and institutions both at the national at **local levels. Examples of** these projects in palliative care are:

- Canadian Palliative Care Association – National
- All Saints Hospital and Sylvia House – Ottawa
- B.C. Children's Hospital – British Columbia
- Dorothy Ley Hospice – Toronto
- Kairos House – Edmonton
- Manitoba Hospice Foundation – Manitoba
- Pain control research – Calgary
- Palliative Care Projects in Atlantic Canada – Acadia
- Palliative Care Units at Royal Victoria Hospital and **Hopital** Notre Dame de la Merci – Montréal

The Calgary and Edmonton Commanderies are pleased to have supported the development and publication of A Caregiver's Guide.

THE MILITARY AND HOSPITALLER ORDER OF ST. LAZARUS OF JERUSALEM

INDEX

D

E

F

G

H

I

L

M

N

O

P

R

S

NOTES FOR YOU AND YOUR NURSE